GERM CELL TUMOR

Edited by **Angabin Matin**

Germ Cell Tumor
Edited by Angabin Matin

Published by InTech
Janeza Trdine 9, 51000 Rijeka, Croatia

Publishing Process Manager Dragana Manestar

Technical Editor Teodora Smiljanic

Cover Designer InTech Design Team

Additional hard copies can be obtained from orders@intechopen.com

Germ Cell Tumor, Edited by Angabin Matin
p. cm.
ISBN 978-953-51-0456-8

For EU product safety concerns:
IN TECH d.o.o., Prolaz Marije Krucifikse Kozulić 3, 51000 Rijeka, Croatia,
info@intechopen.com or visit our website at intechopen.com.

Meet the editor

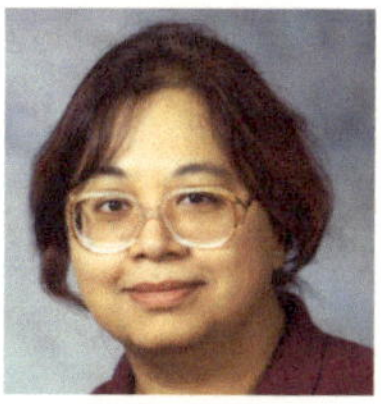

Dr. Angabin Matin is an Associate Professor in the Department of Genetics at MD Anderson Cancer Center in Houston, Texas. She received her Bachelor and Master of Science degrees from the University of Singapore. She obtained her Ph.D. in 1993 in Cancer Biology from the Graduate School of Biomedical Sciences at Houston, University of Texas, USA. Her current research focuses on using mouse models to dissect the complex genetic causes underlying testicular germ cell tumor development. Together with collaborators, her laboratory identified that loss of the RNA binding protein, DND1, predisposes mice to develop testicular germ cell tumors. There is growing interest to understand the biological role of DND1, a novel regulator of translation, both in normal germ cells and in germ cell tumors. Her laboratory is also involved in mapping and identifying novel testicular tumor predisposing loci and genes in mice.

Contents

Preface

In Germ Cell Tumor, leading scientists and physicians from different countries have contributed to review the latest ideas and developments regarding the clinical presentation, current treatment modalities and the biology and genetics of germ cell tumors. Most authors have focused on testicular germ cell tumors which are the most common cancers in young adult males and whose incidence has been increasing in recent years.

The book is divided into two sections. The first section, Clinical Perspectives, discusses observations and current ideas regarding presentation and treatment of germ cell tumors in children and adults. Clinical perspectives includes a comprehensive review by Nick Liu and co-authors regarding the pathogenesis, risk factors, diagnosis and treatment regimens applied to intratubular germ cell neoplasia which are the precursor, pre-invasive lesion for testicular cancers. In Chapter 2, Paul Johnston and Stephen Beck review current management options for the most common type of germ cell tumors of the testes, non-seminomatous germ cell tumors. In Chapter 3, Takamitsu Fujimaki reviews intracranial germ cell tumors, which affect mostly children, and their diagnosis and treatment. Additionally, Chapter 4 reviews current management strategies for all the different histological sub-types of testicular cancers. Nikhil Vasdev and Andrew Thorpe provide a European perspective on treatment of germ cell tumors.

In the second section, Scientific Perspectives, the chapters review current perspectives on experimental systems such as mouse models of testicular germ cell tumors and the genetics and epigenetics of germ cell tumor development in humans and in mice. Delphine Carouge and Joseph Nadeau provide a thorough review on mouse models of testicular germ cell tumors (Chapter 6). They also compare results obtained from genetic studies of testicular cancer susceptibility in humans to that in mice. Epigenetic dysregulation is implicated in a variety of cancers, including in testicular cancers. Christopher Payne presents an up to date review on the epigenetic modifications found in normal germ cells, in the pre-invasive precursor cells and in testicular germ cell tumors of young adults (Chapter 7). Yiermi Soini reviews the role of claudins, which are components of tight junctions, in germ cell tumors (Chapter 8).

These chapters will be useful for scientists, physicians and lay readers wishing to review the current status of our knowledge regarding germ cell cancers. We hope that the chapters will serve to inspire further ideas towards increased understanding of development of germ cell cancers and improved treatment and management of this disease. I thank all the authors for their contributions. In addition, I thank Ms. Gorana Scerbe and Dragana Manestar for their invaluable assistance in the preparation and publication of this book.

Angabin Matin
U.T. M.D. Anderson Cancer Center, Houston, Texas
USA

Part 1

Clinical Perspectives

1

Intratubular Germ Cell Neoplasms of the Testis and Bilateral Testicular Tumors: Clinical Significance and Management Options

Nick W. Liu, Michael C. Risk and Timothy A. Masterson
Department of Urology, Indiana University School of Medicine
Indianapolis,
Indiana
USA

1. Introduction

Although rare, testicular cancer is the most common solid tumor in men between ages 20 and 34, with approximately 5.5 new cases per 100,000 men reported in the United States each year (Howlader et al., 2011). For reasons that are still unclear, the incidence of testicular cancer worldwide has doubled in the past 40 years, with the most significant increases seen in industrialized countries in North America, Europe and Oceania (Huyghe et al., 2003). The vast majority of malignant testicular tumors are testicular germ cell tumors (TGCTs), which can be divided into two main categories: seminomas and non-seminomas. The pathogenesis of TGCTs has been the subject of intense interest recently due to the rising incidence (Chia et al., 2010). Skakkebaek was the first to describe the possibility of a pre-invasive lesion for testicular cancer in 1972, when he identified atypical germ cells in the testes of two infertile men who later developed TGCTs (Skakkebaek, 1972). Subsequent work by Skakkebaek et al. confirmed the existence of a precursor lesion for TGCTs. Historically, the terms carcinoma in situ and testicular intraepithelial neoplasia have been used to describe this lesion, but they are no longer preferred because these lesions do not possess epithelial features (Emerson & Ulbright, 2010). The preferred term used in recent literature, including this review, is intratubular germ cell neoplasia, unclassified (ITGCN).

ITCGN plays an important role in the development of TGCTs. Since the seminal work by Skakkebaek, it has been generally accepted that most TGCTs arise from ITGCN, with the notable exception of pediatric germ cell tumors (yolk sac, mature teratoma) and the rare spermatocytic seminomas. Subsequent work by von der Maase et al. demonstrated that patients with ITGCN will ultimately progress to invasive cancer if left untreated(von der Maase et al., 1986). This malignant transformation has led researchers to focus on early detection and treatment in order to improve the outcomes in testicular cancer. Advances in molecular biology have helped us gain insight into the mechanisms involved in the transformation of ITGCN to TGCTs. In this chapter, we will focus on the pathogenesis, risk factors, diagnosis and treatment regimens utilized in the management of ITGCN and bilateral TGCTs.

2. Pathogenesis

A close association between seminoma and non-seminoma was described long before the discovery of ITGCN (Akhtar & Sidiki, 1979; Mark & Hedinger, 1965). Numerous studies have since demonstrated that both histologies can often co-exist in the same tumor and share similar risk factors, hinting toward a common etiopathogenesis (Bray et al., 2006). The likelihood of common origin has also been supported by epidemiological studies. When analyzing the testicular cancer incidence between 1973 and 2002, Chia and colleagues found the incidence trends of seminoma and non-seminoma were similar to each other suggesting common risk factors (Chia et al., 2010). In contrast, these trends were not observed in those with pediatric testicular cancer, indicating different inciting factors are involved in this population (Lacerda et al., 2009). Histologic studies on orchiectomy specimens taken from patients with TGCTs also confirmed the high incidence of a common precursor lesion associated with both seminoma and non-seminoma. Following his initial description of ITGCN in 1972, Skakkebaek identified ITGCN in 77% of orchiectomy specimens taken from patients with seminoma, embryonal carcinoma or terato-carcinoma (Skakkebaek, 1975). ITGCN has also been found in as many as 98% of orchiectomy specimens containing both seminoma and non-seminoma (Jacobsen et al., 1981). Interestingly, while the majority of patients with ITGCN undoubtedly progress to TGCTs, those without evidence of ITGCN tend not to develop invasive testicular tumors (von der Maase et al., 1986). This finding lends support to the concept that ITGCN serves as the initial gateway to TGCTs.

A strong connection between ITGCN and TGCTs can be realized through two large autopsies studies from Europe, which demonstrated similar prevalence of ITGCN to lifetime risk of TGCTs (Giwercman et al., 1991a; Linke et al., 2005). Subsequent studies on infertile men with untreated ITGCN found that many will progress to invasive tumors, with risk approaching 70% at 7 years (von der Maase et al., 1986). There is strong evidence suggesting that ITGCN is present years prior to development of overt cancer. Muller and colleagues followed a 10 year-old cryptorchid boy with repeated testicular biopsies, which showed ITGCN at age 13 and eventually invasive malignant growth at age 21 (Muller et al., 1984; Skakkebaek et al., 1987). This idea was further supported by the morphological similarity between ITGCN and human fetal gonocytes observed by Holstein and Korner in 1974 (Holstein & Korner, 1974). Through immunohistochemical and DNA studies, Jorgense and colleagues were able to support their hypothesis that ITGCN cells are of prenatal origin and may be a consequence of malignant transformation of fetal germ cells *in utero* (Jorgensen et al., 1993).

Histologic and molecular studies have provided strong evidence supporting the close association between ITGCN and TGCTs. Due to its high serum concentration in seminoma patients, placental-like alkaline phosphatase (PLAP), a molecule of unknown biological function, was one of the first tumor markers studied for testicular cancer (Jacobsen & Norgaard-Pedersen, 1984). Through immunohistochemical experiments, PLAP was found to be highly expressed in seminomas, embryonal carcinomas, and ITGCN(Manivel et al., 1987). In contrast, expression of PLAP was not observed in normal testicular tissues (Manivel et al., 1987). As a result of recent advances in molecular pathology, numerous markers specific for ITCGN and TGCTs have been discovered. These markers include M2A (Giwercman et al., 1988a), 49-3F (Giwercman et al., 1990b), TRA-1-60 (Giwercman et al., 1993a), NANOG (Hart et al., 2005; Hoei-Hansen et al., 2005a), *c-kit* (Rajpert-De Meyts & Skakkebaek, 1994), AP-2y (Hoei-Hansen et al., 2004b), and OCT 3/4 (de Jong et al., 2005; Jones et al., 2006). Detailed discussion of these markers is beyond the scope of this chapter, but some of them deserve further mention here. *c-kit* is a cell membrane tyrosine kinase receptor responsible for migration and survival of primordial germ cells. Its expression is seen in both ITGCN and seminoma. Mutations in the *c-kit* gene are frequently encountered in patients with bilateral germ cell tumors but rare in those with unilateral disease (Rajpert-De Meyts, 2006). This finding suggests that mutations had occurred prior to migration of primordial germ cells early in life and patients with *c-kit* mutations are prone to develop bilateral germ cell tumors. Recently, OCT3/4 has become one of the most widely used germ cell tumor markers due to its high specificity and sensitivity for seminoma, embryonal carcinoma and ITGCN (Jones et al., 2006). OCT3/4 has been praised as a possible screening tool for patients at risk for the development of TGCTs (Cheng et al., 2007; Jones et al., 2006).

The exact mechanisms involved in the transformation of ITGCN to overt TGCTs are not well understood, partly due to the lack of good experimental and animal models (Hoei-Hansen et al., 2005b). Down regulation of PTEN and p18 expressions as well as induction of cyclin E have been implicated in the progression of ITGCN to invasive tumors (Bartkova et al., 2000; Di Vizio et al., 2005). Through comparative genomic analysis, Summersgill and colleagues were able to show that the gain of chromosome 12p, a consistent finding in TGCTs, is associated with survival of ITGCN independent of Sertoli cells leading to malignant transformation (Looijenga et al., 2003; Summersgill et al., 2001). While there is strong evidence indicating ITGCN is the precursor for all TGCTs, the question still remains: where does ITGCN come from? The most widely accepted hypothesis suggests that ITCGN originates from fetal gonocytes and the initiation of malignant transformation most likely takes place early in fetal development. This hypothesis was initially based on the close morphological similarities between ITGCN and fetal gonocytes noted by Skakkebaek as well as other investigators (Gondos et al., 1983; Holstein & Korner, 1974). Subsequent studies demonstrating similar expression patterns between ITGCN, TGCTs and fetal gonoctyes of many immunohistochemical markers lend further support to this hypothesis (Jorgensen et al., 1993). Interestingly, expression of these markers is not seen in the adult testis (Jorgensen et al., 1993). Recent development of high throughput expression technology has not only provided better characterization of gene expressions of ITGCN at the RNA level but also helped us gain further insights into the relationship between ITGCN and fetal gonocytes. By comparing the mRNA expression of ITGCN to normal testis tissue, Hoei-Hansen et al. was the first to focus on the expression pattern of ITGCN and subsequently identified several genes that are important to fetal testicular development (Hoei-Hansen et al., 2004a). In 2004, Almstrup and colleagues used genome-wide cDNA microarrays to compare genomic expression profiles of ITGCN and embryonic stem cells, a precursor to fetal gonocytes, and found a remarkable similarity in expression patterns between these two entities, providing additional support that ITGCN is of fetal origin (Almstrup et al., 2004). Similar conclusions have been reached by other investigators as well. A recent microarray analysis by Sonne et al. demonstrated that the expression patterns of ITGCN cells are more similar to those of gonocyte than embryonic stem cells, suggesting that ITGCN may simply be an arrested gonocyte that persisted in a postnatal testis (Sonne et al., 2009).

Two mechanisms regarding the development of ITGCN can be proposed based on the current discussion. Whether the formation of ITGCN is related to spontaneous regression of spermatogonia toward a primordial germ cell state or an abnormal persistence of an arrested gonocyte beyond the neonatal period remains unanswered. Some researchers have attempted to address this through epidemiologic studies by specifically examining the correlation between cancer incidence and differences in environmental factors during time of fetal development and birth. Moller's work in 1989 demonstrated lower incidence of testicular cancer in men born around the time of World War II than expected from the overall increasing trend. His observation supports the hypothesis that environmental influences early in life, or *in utero*, may be the determining factor for testicular cancer development (Moller, 1989; 1993). Additional evidence supporting this hypothesis can be seen in two cohort studies from Denmark, a country known to have one of the highest incidences of testicular cancer. By looking at the incidence of testicular cancer according to residence at birth within Denmark, Myrup et al was able to show the risk for TGCTs is related to county of birth, rather than county of residence at diagnosis (Myrup et al., 2010). When evaluating the testicular cancer risk in first- and second-generation immigrants to Denmark, it was found that the first-generation immigrants have TGCT risk similar to their country of origin, whereas the second generation has a risk similar to the Danish incidence (Myrup et al., 2008). Similar results have been produced by investigators from Sweden as well (Hemminki & Li, 2002). All of the evidence presented thus far would argue that the fate of testicular cancer is determined early in life, and the transformation of a precursor cell to ITGCN is initiated during fetal development.

3. Risk factors

Since ITGCN is a precursor lesion for TGCTs, the presence of ITGCN is now recognized as a risk factor for TGCTs. However, the incidence of ITGCN in healthy men has not been well characterized as the diagnosis of ITGCN requires testicular biopsy. As mentioned earlier, two landmark pathological studies attempted to address this question. The researchers from Denmark analyzed 399 testes from men between age 18 to 50 years old who died unexpectedly and found the overall prevalence of ITGCN to be 0.8%, comparable to the lifetime risk of TGCTs in the Danish male population (Giwercman et al., 1991a). The autopsy study from Germany also demonstrated similar findings (Linke et al., 2005). A number of conditions with high prevalence of ITGCN haven been identified and will be discussed here.

One of the greatest risk factors for developing TGCTs is a personal history of TGCTs. It has been shown that patients with a personal history of testicular cancer have a 25-fold increased risk of developing TGCTs in the contralateral testis (Dieckmann et al., 1993). Studies on men with TGCTs who underwent contralateral testicular biopsy demonstrated consistent rates of ITGCN at around 5-7% (Berthelsen et al., 1982; Dieckmann & Loy, 1996; von der Maase et al., 1986). Once again, the prevalence of ITGCN in the contralateral testis correlates well with the lifetime risk of developing contralateral TGCTs (Grigor & Rorth, 1993; von der Maase et al., 1986). Additional studies on men with unilateral TGCTs have identified a number of risk factors associated with contralateral ITGCN. Several reports have demonstrated testicular atrophy as an independent risk factor for contralateral ITCGN, with 4.3-fold increased risk of having positive biopsies in this group of patients (Dieckmann & Loy, 1996; Harland et al., 1998). Age at presentation is also a concern for contralateral ITGCN. One study showed that diagnosis of TGCTs in patients younger than 30 is associated with significant increased risk of positive biopsies on the contralateral testes

(Harland et al., 1998). While these findings demonstrate testicular atrophy and age of presentation are both strong risk factors for ITGCN, it has also been shown that the majority of patients with ITGCN do not have these associated risk factors. A large portion of patients with ITGCN would be missed if contralateral biopsies were only performed in patients with these risk factors. Dieckmann et al. have advocated for performing biopsies in all men with a history of testicular cancer (Dieckmann & Skakkebaek, 1999). In addition to atrophy and age of presentation, an irregular echogenic pattern of the contralateral testis on ultrasound has been shown to be predictive of positive testicular biopsy for ITGCN in 78 men with unilateral TGCTs (Lenz et al., 1996).

A recent study of 22,562 men in the US demonstrated that infertility is a strong risk factor for testicular cancer, suggesting that infertility and testicular cancer share a common etiology (Walsh et al., 2009). Similar findings were observed in a study of 2739 patients who underwent testicular biopsy for infertility (Bettocchi et al., 1994). In this cohort, 16 patients had unilateral ITGCN and testicular atrophy, 50% progressed to invasive TGCTs. Previous studies have shown that the incidence of ITGCN in infertile men is about 0.4-1.1% (Pryor et al., 1983; Skakkebaek, 1978). A recent retrospective review of biopsies from 453 subfertile men revealed a 2.2% risk of ITGCN, compared to an estimated risk of 0.45% in an age- and birth-matched cohort, suggesting that infertility is a risk factor for ITGCN (Olesen et al., 2007). In agreement with previous findings, these authors concluded that severe oligospermia and atrophic testes are associated risks for ITGCN.

Patients with cryptorchidism or undescended testes (UDT) are at an increased risk for developing testicular cancer. A recent meta-analysis review of 11 studies demonstrated that men with UDT are at a 6.3-fold increased risk for TGCTs, compared to 1.7-fold increase in the unaffected testes (Akre et al., 2009). Furthermore, there is strong evidence suggesting that orchiopexy before puberty has a protective effect against development of testicular cancer (Wood & Elder, 2009). While there is convincing evidence linking cryptorchidism to testicular cancer, the relationship between UDT and prevalence of ITGCN remains unclear. An early biopsy study on 50 men with cryptorchidism demonstrated the prevalence of ITGCN in this cohort is around 8% (Krabbe et al., 1979). In contrast, a larger study involving 300 patients with UDT found the prevalence of ITGCN to be 1.7% (Giwercman et al., 1989). Furthermore, previous studies on the prevalence of ITGCN in patients with unilateral TCGTs found that history of cryptorchidism is not predictive of ITGCN (Dieckmann & Loy, 1996; Harland et al., 1993). Unlike cryptorchidism, patients with sexual developmental disorders have been shown to have high rates of ITGCN and TGCTs in several small studies (Skakkebaek, 1979; Slowikowska-Hilczer et al., 2001).

Significant controversy surrounds the association between testicular microlithiasis (TM) and the subsequent development of ITCGN and TGCTs. In an otherwise healthy population, TM is not considered a risk factor for TGCTs. One study involving 63 healthy men with TM demonstrated that 98.5% of this cohort remained cancer-free 5 years after the initial screening (DeCastro et al., 2008). Furthermore, the incidence of TM in asymptomatic young men is reportedly to be 1.5-5.6% (DeCastro et al., 2008; von Eckardstein et al., 2001). On the other hand, the association between TM and TGCTs is also well documented, with high incidence of TM observed in patients with testicular cancer (Ikinger et al., 1982; Sanli et al., 2008). Recently, a large meta-analysis attempted to address this issue by looking at the association of TM with TGCT and ITGCN (Tan et al., 2010). The authors found no association between TM and increased risk of TCGT in the otherwise healthy males. However, in those patients at risk for TGCTs, such as infertility, UDT or history of unilateral TGCT, the presence of TM is associated with approximately a 10-fold increased risk for concurrent diagnosis of TGCT or ITGCN. These findings are in an agreement with previous studies as well. Holm et al. demonstrated the presence of TM in the contralateral testis of men with unilateral TGCTs is associated with about a 30-fold increased risk of ITGCN (Holm et al., 2003). Furthermore, the incidence of TM in infertile men has been shown to be 2-20%, which is considerably higher than that of the general population (de Gouveia Brazao et al., 2004; von Eckardstein et al., 2001). Others have suggested that bilateral microlithiasis and sonographic heterogeneity in subfertile men are associated with increased risk of developing ITGCN (de Gouveia Brazao et al., 2004; Elzinga-Tinke et al., 2010), indicating the need to follow these patients closely with frequent biopsy or ultrasound.

4. Diagnosis

There are no imaging modalities or serum tumor markers to accurately diagnose ITGCN. Currently, testicular biopsy is the only reliable method to diagnose ITGCN. The pathologic morphology of ITGCN is well-defined and is similar to that of seminoma. The ITGCN cells are larger than normal spermatogonia, and possess larger nuclei with prominent nucleoli (Gondos & Migliozzi, 1987). The cytoplasm is rich with glycogen and contains the enzyme PLAP (Dieckmann et al., 2011; Lauke, 1997). These abnormal cells are located at the basement membrane of the seminiferous tubules and the tubules vary from containing adjacent normal Sertoli cells and spermatogonia to complete dominance of ITGCN cells (Jacobsen et al., 1981). A good biopsy sample should be at least 3 x 3 mm in size and contains at least 30-40 tubules on microscopic examination (Holstein & Lauke, 1996). Testicular biopsies should be placed in Boulin's or Stieve's solution; Formalin fixation should be avoided because it can greatly alter the morphology of testicular architecture.

Immunohistochemical markers are routinely used during histological examination to aid the diagnosis of ITGCN. The importance of immunohistochemistry (IHC) was highlighted in a recent review of 20 patients with TGCTs and prior negative testicular biopsy (van Casteren et al., 2009). Seven cases of ITGCNs and TGCTs were diagnosed by experienced pathologists based on morphology alone, but an additional 4 cases were identified with IHC. As mentioned earlier, PLAP has traditionally been the most widely used IHC marker to identify ITGCN, with sensitivity ranging from 83-98% (Jacobsen & Norgaard-Pedersen, 1984; Manivel et al., 1987). Several studies recently have demonstrated a superior IHC marker for detecting ITGCN, OCT3/4, which has sensitivity and specificity approaching 100% (Cheng et al., 2007; de Jong et al., 2005; Jones et al., 2006). A pathologic representation of ITGCN stained with OCT 3/4 is portrayed in Fig. 1.

As open testicular biopsy is invasive and has the potential for complications, detection of ITGCN by semen analysis has been investigated. The ability to use semen to detect ITGCN is based on the original work by Giwercman when he observed the exfoliation of ITGCN cells from the seminiferous tubules into the seminal fluid in men with TGCTs (Giwercman et al., 1988b). However, the detection rate of ITGCN cells in semen is far inferior to open surgical biopsy (Brackenbury et al., 1993). Subsequent studies have attempted to increase the sensitivity of semen analysis for CIS by combining DNA flow cytometry and in situ hybridization without great success (Giwercman et al., 1990a). Recently, investigators from Denmark sought to improve the detection rate on semen analysis by developing a sophisticated model involving immunocytochemical staining of ejaculates from infertile men (Almstrup et al., 2011). This approach demonstrated an overall sensitivity and specificity of 0.67 and 0.98, respectively, when compared to open surgical biopsy. These non-invasive methods for detection of ITGCN are promising but their clinical feasibility remains to be seen.

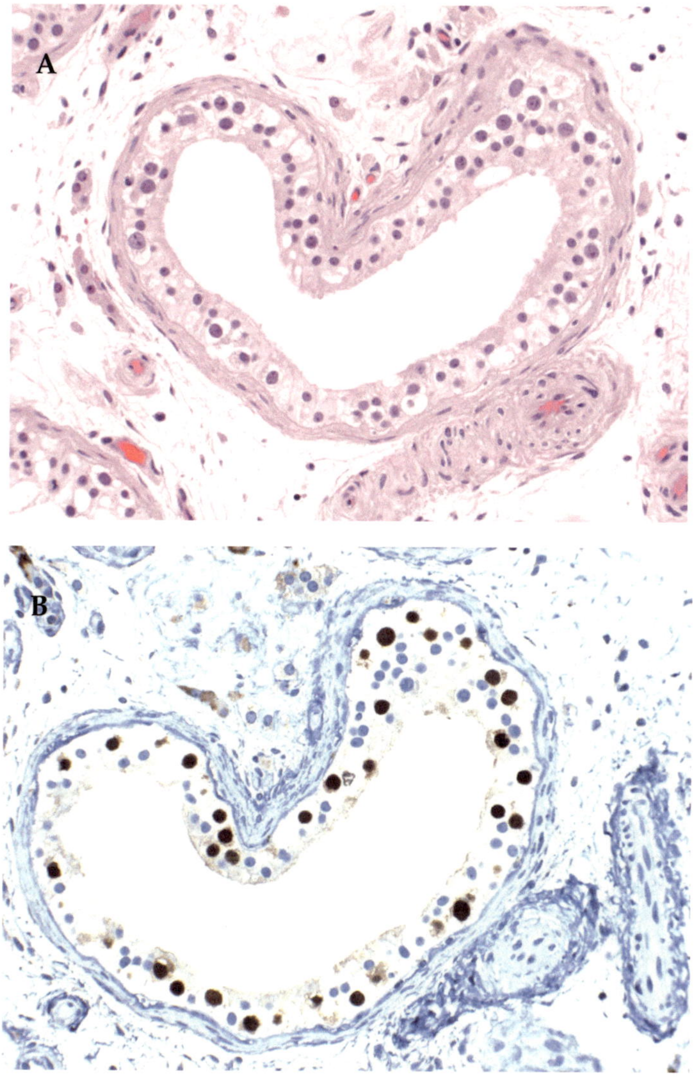

Fig. 1. Pathologic features of ITGCN. A – H&E stained section demonstrates typical features of ITGCN: cells with large nuclei and prominent nucleoli located along the basement membrane of the seminiferous tubules. B – Immunohistochemical staining of ITGCN cells with OCT 4 demonstrating a nuclear staining pattern (Jones et al., 2004). (Courtesy of Liang Cheng, MD, Indiana University School of Medicine, Indianapolis, IN)

4.1 Testicular biopsy

The distribution of ITGCN cells within a testis has been a subject of contention and is directly linked to the accuracy of testicular biopsy. Based on their biopsy simulation experiments, Berthelsen and Skakkebaek hypothesized that ITGCN cells are homogenously dispersed throughout the testis and demonstrated that a 3-mm biopsy is a sufficient representation of the entire testis (Berthelsen & Skakkebaek, 1981). Early studies had supported this theory by demonstrating the low false-negative biopsy rates associated with the single biopsy technique. In a study involving 1859 negative testicular biopsies in the contralateral testes of patients with TGCTs, only 5 patients (0.3%) developed TGCTs (Dieckmann & Loy, 2003). The same authors re-examined their data recently and, again, showed the overall proportion of false-negative biopsies for detecting ITCGN is about 0.5% (Dieckmann et al., 2005). Some investigators have sought to improve the sensitivity of testicular biopsy by performing multiple biopsies on the same testis. In a series of 2318 men with TGCTs who underwent double-biopsy of the contralateral testes, the discordance rate was 31% with an extra yield of 18% in diagnosis (Dieckmann et al., 2007). The high discordance rate in this study suggests that the distribution of ITGCN within a testis is heterogeneous rather than homogenous. This finding is further supported by several ITGCN mapping studies that demonstrated a focal pattern of ITGCN adjacent to TGCTs (Loy et al., 1990; Prym & Lauke, 1994). The heterogeneous distribution of ITGCN would also provide an explanation for the development of TGCTs despite prior negative biopsies. Based on this assumption, Dieckmann and colleagues were able to increase the diagnostic yield of ITGCN by performing a second biopsy at a different site (Dieckmann et al., 2007). This is in accord with a study involving triple biopsies of the contralateral testis, which demonstrated an 8% increase in detection of ITGCN (Kliesch et al., 2003). However, this approach may result in a higher complication rate especially in the setting of a solitary testis. Furthermore, it remains to be seen whether the benefit of multiple biopsies outweighs its risks. Even with this approach subsequent TGCTs in patients with prior negative double biopsy have been reported (Souchon et al., 2006).

Complications associated with testicular biopsy remain a major concern and have prevented many clinicians from adopting this approach as routine screening protocol. Current literature suggests the overall rates of complication secondary to testicular biopsy range from 3 - 20% (Dieckmann et al., 2005; Heidenreich & Moul, 2002). In a prospective study of 1874 men with testicular cancer who underwent contralateral testicular biopsy, the overall complication rate of 2.8% was noted with 0.64% requiring repeat surgery and one testis (0.05%) was lost (Dieckmann et al., 2005). In the same series, a subset of patients were followed with serial scrotal sonographic and magnetic resonance imaging, which demonstrated early post-operative changes, such as hematoma or edema, in 33% - 45% of patients. However, these changes spontaneously resolved in 96% of patients 18 months after the initial biopsy, suggesting testicular biopsy is a procedure with low-surgical risks. Despite resolution of post-surgical changes on imaging, the impact of surgical biopsy on testicular endocrine function remains to be addressed in this cohort of patients. Studies on infertile men have reported decrease in serum testosterone level following testicular biopsy, with some developing hypogonadism (Manning et al., 1998); however, these cases were done with significantly more biopsies per testis and the effect was self-limiting.

The question of which group of patients should undergo testicular biopsy has been a subject of controversy, with varying responses to the same data. The fundamental argument for routine testicular biopsy is early diagnosis of TGCTs at the precursor stages. The most common scenario in which testicular biopsy is performed to detect ITGCN is in the contralateral testes of patients with a history of unilateral TGCTs. Surgical biopsy of the contralateral testis at the time of initial orchiectomy is routinely done in Denmark and Germany, two counties with the world's highest incidences of TGCTs (Dieckmann et al., 2011). Others have advocated for biopsy only in those with TGCTs and risk factors for contralateral ITGCN, such as testicular atrophy, history of cryptorchidism, age less than 30 years, infertility and TM (Dieckmann et al., 2011; Heidenreich, 2009). As demonstrated earlier, those who routinely perform testicular biopsy have consistently demonstrated a 5-7% incidence rate of ITGCN in the contralateral testis, and 70% of them progress to TGCTs at 7 years (Dieckmann & Loy, 1996; von der Maase et al., 1986). Early identification of these high risk patients allows for organ-sparing therapy, which may potentially preserve endocrine function in contrast to a second orchiectomy (Dieckmann & Skakkebaek, 1999). Additionally, diagnostic delay in patients with TGCTs has been shown to significantly impact survival, which highlights the importance of early diagnosis (Huyghe et al., 2007). Since the rate of false-negative biopsy is exceedingly low (0.5%), a negative testicular biopsy translates into a very low probability of having a second TGCTs. This may dictate a less intensive surveillance protocol as well as alleviate psychological distress associated with diagnosis of cancer in high-risk patients.

The arguments against the practice of routine testicular biopsy in these patients are also convincing. In contrast to the standard of care in Denmark and Germany, physicians in the US are less likely to perform routine testicular biopsy in patients with TGCTs partly due to a lower incidence of contralateral cancer (Coogan et al., 1998; Fossa et al., 2005). In a large series of nearly 30,000 patients with unilateral TGCT, the investigators demonstrated an overall risk of developing contralateral TGCTs is 1.9% in the US (Fossa et al., 2005), which is considerably lower than the 5-7% reported by the European studies. Furthermore, these authors demonstrated patients with contralateral TGCTs had excellent long-term prognosis, with an overall survival rate of 93% at 10 years after initial diagnosis, providing support for continuing the US approach of not subjecting contralateral testis to biopsy. Others have also demonstrated good clinical outcomes in patients with bilateral TGCTs who are treated appropriately for histology and stage (Holzbeierlein et al., 2003). Other arguments favoring the omission of routine biopsy include the added cost associated with surgery as well as exposing the majority of patients unnecessarily to the surgical risks in order to benefit a few individuals. As discussed earlier, testicular biopsy to screen for ITGCN is not a perfect technique; many cases of contralateral tumor occurrence have been reported in patients with negative prior biopsies, even with the double biopsy approach (Souchon et al., 2006). Finally, the most widely accepted organ-sparing therapy for ITGCN is radiotherapy, which has been shown to destroy both endocrine and exocrine function of a testis, with one study demonstrating high incidence of hypogonadisim after radiation requiring androgen supplementation (Petersen et al., 2002). Until methods of diagnosis are improved or a survival benefit is demonstrated with early diagnosis of ITGCN, treatment decisions need to be made based on data presented and individualized for patient risk factors and wishes.

5. Treatment

The primary goal of treating ITCGN is to prevent its malignant transformation to TGCT. Presently, there are four options to managing ITGCN: chemotherapy, radiation, orchiectomy and surveillance. With the exception of surveillance, the remaining three treatment modalities put patients at significant risk for infertility, hypogonadism, or both. The decision to proceed with a certain treatment modality has to be individualized based upon specific risk factors as well as patient wishes.

5.1 Chemotherapy

It was initially thought that chemotherapy could completely eradicate ITGCN and prevent development of contralateral TGCT. This idea was based on the observation that patients receiving chemotherapy had no progression of disease and had complete resolution of ITGCN on repeat biopsy, whereas 7 out of 18 patients without chemotherapy progressed to overt cancer (von der Maase et al., 1985). However, three years after their initial publication, the same investigators reported that one patient in the chemotherapy group had recurrence of ITGCN on repeat biopsy (von der Maase et al., 1988). Numerous reports since then demonstrated chemotherapy to be an ineffective regimen for treating ITGCN. One series estimated the risk of recurrent ITGCN 5 and 10 years after termination of chemotherapy to be 21% and 42%, respectively (Christensen et al., 1998). Histological analysis on orchiectomy specimens obtained from patients who had chemotherapy demonstrated persistence of ITGCN in 35% of patients (Bottomley et al., 1990). Possible explanations behind this phenomenon include the presence of blood-testis barrier or insensitivity of ITGCN cells to chemotherapy (Mortensen et al., 2011; Ploen & Setchell, 1992). In a recent study of 11 patients with unilateral TGCTs and biopsy-proven ITGCN in the contralateral testis treated with chemotherapy, 64% of them had ITGCN on repeat biopsy, providing support that chemotherapy is ineffective at eradicating ITGCN (Kleinschmidt et al., 2009).

5.2 Radical orchiectomy

Unlike chemotherapy, orchiectomy is the most definitive treatment with the highest success rate and is the main treatment approach for three patient populations: those with unilateral ITGCN and contralateral normal testis; those with an atrophic testis; and those with infertility and unilateral ITGCN (Dieckmann & Skakkebaek, 1999; Mortensen et al., 2011). In patients with a solitary testis, orchiectomy in this population needs to be weighed against the risk of infertility and permanent dependence on exogenous testosterone replacement.

5.3 Radiation

Local radiation has become the preferred treatment modality for ITGCN because it is organ-sparing and highly effective at eradicating ITGCN cells. The rationale behind employing radiotherapy is based on the finding that radiation has the propensity to destroy ITGCN and germ cells while preserving Leydig cell function (von der Maase et al., 1985). Therefore, it has the potential of preserving testicular endocrine function while eliminating neoplastic cells. Presently, three major concerns have been raised regarding radiotherapy in the treatment of ITGCN. First, the radiation dose for optimal oncologic control has not been determined (Mortensen et al., 2011). The current recommended dose according to guidelines put forth by the European Association of Urology is 20 Gy delivered over 2 weeks (Albers et al., 2005). This dose has previously been shown to be very effective at eradicating ITGCN cells, with one series demonstrating complete resolution of ITGCN on repeat biopsy at a follow-up of 2 years (Giwercman et al., 1991b). Another group from Denmark studied the effect of radiotherapy in doses 14 to 20 Gy on eradication of ITGCN testes, and demonstrated that all patients treated with radiation dose level 16 to 20 Gy had complete resolution of ITGCN while one patient treated at dose level 14 Gy had a recurrence at a follow up of 5 years (Petersen et al., 2002). However, recurrences of ITGCN have been reported at all dose levels up to 20 Gy (Classen et al., 2003; Dieckmann et al., 2002; Dotsch et al., 2000; Petersen et al., 2002). Currently, there is no consensus on the optimal radiation dose to achieve cancer control, but most would agree that a dose level of 16 to 20 Gy is effective. The second concern is in regards to the effect of radiation on testicular exocrine function. Local radiation to the testis will result in the destruction of both ITGCN and germ cells, subsequently rendering these patients infertile. Proponents of local radiation to solitary testes argue that patients with ITGCN already have severely impaired spermatogensis prior to therapy (Giwercman et al., 1993b; Petersen et al., 1999); therefore, radiation should not have significant impact on the development of infertility. However, improvement in spermatogenesis has been noted following removal of unilateral TGCTs (Carroll et al., 1987) and cases of successful conception in patients with ITGCN have been reported (Heidenreich et al., 1997). Therefore, it is important to consider surveillance or postponing radiation to allow for paternity in patients with ITGCN in the solitary testis. The third concern is the impairment of testicular endocrine function by local radiation. According to one series of patients with ITGCN in solitary testis, serum luteinizing hormone remained significantly elevated post radiation and 25% of patients require permanent androgen supplementation (Giwercman et al., 1991b). This finding led to several investigations on dose reduction, with one study demonstrating the impairment on endocrine function was independent of radiation dose and the need for androgen substitutions was similar at all dose levels (Petersen et al., 2002). Others found less toxic effect on testicular Leydig cell function with lower radiation doses at 13 and 16 Gy (Bang et al., 2009; Sedlmayer et al., 2001). All patients undergoing radiation therapy need to have their hormone function checked on a regular basis in order to identify those where androgen supplementation is needed.

5.4 Active surveillance

For select patients, active surveillance may be the treatment of choice. This is particularly true for those with ITGCN in the solitary testis who desire to preserve fertility and hormone function. Surveillance can be justified in these patients but they must be counseled on the risk of developing invasive cancer and the need for subsequent orchiectomy. Furthermore, these patients need to be compliant with regular follow-up and, more importantly, frequent testicular self-examination. If preserving fertility is the goal, semen analysis should be obtained and cryopreservation of viable sperm should be considered before treatment is initiated (Dieckmann & Skakkebaek, 1999). For those patients who progress to TGCTs, partial orchiectomy may be an acceptable treatment if the tumor is organ-confined and less than 2cm in size (Heidenreich et al., 2001). Consistent with the discussion above, as most patients in this series (82%) had associated ITGCN, most were treated with adjuvant radiation and relapses were only observed in those who did not receive radiation treatment. Partial orchiectomy is still in the investigational phase, and patients should be counseled on the risk of disease progression and the need for radical orchiectomy if a tumor recurs in that testis.

6. Bilateral testicular cancer

While the risk of developing contralateral testicular cancer is high in patients with unilateral TGCTs, there is no clear consensus on how these patients should be managed. Perhaps, we can gain further insight into this issue by looking at the outcome data of patients with bilateral testicular cancer. The reported incidence of bilateral TGCTs in the US and Europe is estimated to be 1- 4% (Bokemeyer et al., 1993; Che et al., 2002; Coogan et al., 1998; Fossa et al., 2005; Hentrich et al., 2005; Holzbeierlein et al., 2003; Pamenter et al., 2003). In these contemporary series, metachronous presentations were the majority (62-88%) and the median interval between first and second testicular tumor was 50 – 76 months. Recent studies demonstrated that the clinical outcomes of metachronous TGCTs were excellent (Albers et al., 1999; Che et al., 2002; Coogan et al., 1998; Fossa et al., 2005), with the majority of patients presenting with clinical stage 1 disease (44 – 90%). Furthermore, the 10-year survival rate following a diagnosis of metachronous bilateral testis cancer was 93%, which is comparable to patients diagnosed with unilateral TGCTs (95%)(Fossa et al., 2005). Single institution studies from Indiana, M.D. Anderson, and Memorial-Sloan-Kettering also demonstrated excellent prognosis in these patients, with most reporting very low mortality from TGCTs (Che et al., 2002; Coogan et al., 1998; Holzbeierlein et al., 2003). Despite such a high cure rate, most patients in these studies did not undergo contralateral testicular biopsy. This finding certainly questions the value of contralateral testicular biopsy to screen for ITGCN. Based on the excellent outcomes observed in bilateral TGCTs, active surveillance, perhaps, should play an important role in the management of patients with contralateral ITGCN.

7. Conclusions

The incidence of testicular cancer is increasing worldwide and it has nearly doubled in the last 40 years. This increasing incidence has led researchers to focus on the pathogenesis of ITGCN, which has now been established as the precursor lesion for most TGCTs. Several theories have been proposed regarding the origin of ITGCN, and recent studies seem to suggest it is abnormal persistence of an arrested gonocyte beyond the neonatal period. The fate of testicular cancer is determined early in life, and the transformation of a precursor cell to ITGCN cell is initiated *in utero*. Incidence trends of testicular cancer can potentially be altered by continued exploration of the contributing factors in the pre- and peri-natal period. The diagnosis and management of patients with ITGCN remain a challenging problem for clinicians, and indications for testicular biopsy to detect ITGCN are controversial. The decision to proceed with a certain treatment modality should be individualized and needs to be based on specific risk factors as well as patient wishes. Radical orchiectomy and radiation therapy are the only two effective means of preventing subsequent TGCTs in a testis with ITGCN. Both treatment options can result in infertility as well as hormone dysfunction. Metachronous bilateral TGCTs occur infrequently but the clinical outcomes are excellent, suggesting that the role of active surveillance needs to be emphasized in the management of contralateral ITGCN in a solitary testis.

8. References

Akhtar, M. & Sidiki, Y. (1979). "Undifferentiated intratubular germ cell tumor of the testis: light and electron microscopic study of a unique case." Cancer 43(6): 2332-2339.

Akre, O., Pettersson, A. & Richiardi, L. (2009). "Risk of contralateral testicular cancer among men with unilaterally undescended testis: a meta analysis." Int J Cancer 124(3): 687-689.

Albers, P., Albrecht, W., Algaba, F., Bokemeyer, C., Cohn-Cedermark, G., Horwich, A., Klepp, O., Laguna, M. P. & Pizzocaro, G. (2005). "Guidelines on testicular cancer." Eur Urol 48(6): 885-894.

Albers, P., Goll, A., Bierhoff, E., Schoeneich, G. & Muller, S. C. (1999). "Clinical course and histopathologic risk factor assessment in patients with bilateral testicular germ cell tumors." Urology 54(4): 714-718.

Almstrup, K., Hoei-Hansen, C. E., Wirkner, U., Blake, J., Schwager, C., Ansorge, W., Nielsen, J. E., Skakkebaek, N. E., Rajpert-De Meyts, E. & Leffers, H. (2004). "Embryonic stem cell-like features of testicular carcinoma in situ revealed by genome-wide gene expression profiling." Cancer Res 64(14): 4736-4743.

Almstrup, K., Lippert, M., Mogensen, H. O., Nielsen, J. E., Hansen, J. D., Daugaard, G., Jorgensen, N., Foged, N. T., Skakkebaek, N. E. & Rajpert-De Meyts, E. (2011). "Screening of subfertile men for testicular carcinoma in situ by an automated image analysis-based cytological test of the ejaculate." Int J Androl 34(4 Pt 2): e21-30; discussion e30-21.

Bang, A. K., Petersen, J. H., Petersen, P. M., Andersson, A. M., Daugaard, G. & Jorgensen, N. (2009). "Testosterone production is better preserved after 16 than 20 Gray irradiation treatment against testicular carcinoma in situ cells." Int J Radiat Oncol Biol Phys 75(3): 672-676.

Bartkova, J., Thullberg, M., Rajpert-De Meyts, E., Skakkebaek, N. E. & Bartek, J. (2000). "Cell cycle regulators in testicular cancer: loss of p18INK4C marks progression from carcinoma in situ to invasive germ cell tumours." Int J Cancer 85(3): 370-375.

Berthelsen, J. G. & Skakkebaek, N. E. (1981). "Value of testicular biopsy in diagnosing carcinoma in situ testis." Scand J Urol Nephrol 15(3): 165-168.

Berthelsen, J. G., Skakkebaek, N. E., von der Maase, H., Sorensen, B. L. & Mogensen, P. (1982). "Screening for carcinoma in situ of the contralateral testis in patients with germinal testicular cancer." Br Med J (Clin Res Ed) 285(6356): 1683-1686.

Bettocchi, C., Coker, C. B., Deacon, J., Parkinson, C. & Pryor, J. P. (1994). "A review of testicular intratubular germ cell neoplasia in infertile men." J Androl 15 Suppl: 14S-16S.

Bokemeyer, C., Schmoll, H. J., Schoffski, P., Harstrick, A., Bading, M. & Poliwoda, H. (1993). "Bilateral testicular tumours: prevalence and clinical implications." Eur J Cancer 29A(6): 874-876.

Bottomley, D., Fisher, C., Hendry, W. F. & Horwich, A. (1990). "Persistent carcinoma in situ of the testis after chemotherapy for advanced testicular germ cell tumours." Br J Urol 66(4): 420-424.

Brackenbury, E. T., Hargreave, T. B., Howard, G. C. & McIntyre, M. A. (1993). "Seminal fluid analysis and fine-needle aspiration cytology in the diagnosis of carcinoma in situ of the testis." Eur Urol 23(1): 123-128.

Bray, F., Ferlay, J., Devesa, S. S., McGlynn, K. A. & Moller, H. (2006). "Interpreting the international trends in testicular seminoma and nonseminoma incidence." Nat Clin Pract Urol 3(10): 532-543.

Carroll, P. R., Whitmore, W. F., Jr., Herr, H. W., Morse, M. J., Sogani, P. C., Bajorunas, D., Fair, W. R. & Chaganti, R. S. (1987). "Endocrine and exocrine profiles of men with testicular tumors before orchiectomy." J Urol 137(3): 420-423.

Che, M., Tamboli, P., Ro, J. Y., Park, D. S., Ro, J. S., Amato, R. J. & Ayala, A. G. (2002). "Bilateral testicular germ cell tumors: twenty-year experience at M. D. Anderson Cancer Center." Cancer 95(6): 1228-1233.

Cheng, L., Sung, M. T., Cossu-Rocca, P., Jones, T. D., MacLennan, G. T., De Jong, J., Lopez-Beltran, A., Montironi, R. & Looijenga, L. H. (2007). "OCT4: biological functions and clinical applications as a marker of germ cell neoplasia." J Pathol 211(1): 1-9.

Chia, V. M., Quraishi, S. M., Devesa, S. S., Purdue, M. P., Cook, M. B. & McGlynn, K. A. (2010). "International trends in the incidence of testicular cancer, 1973-2002." Cancer Epidemiol Biomarkers Prev 19(5): 1151-1159.

Christensen, T. B., Daugaard, G., Geertsen, P. F. & von der Maase, H. (1998). "Effect of chemotherapy on carcinoma in situ of the testis." Ann Oncol 9(6): 657-660.

Classen, J., Dieckmann, K., Bamberg, M., Souchon, R., Kliesch, S., Kuehn, M. & Loy, V. (2003). "Radiotherapy with 16 Gy may fail to eradicate testicular intraepithelial neoplasia: preliminary communication of a dose-reduction trial of the German Testicular Cancer Study Group." Br J Cancer 88(6): 828-831.

Coogan, C. L., Foster, R. S., Simmons, G. R., Tognoni, P. G., Roth, B. J. & Donohue, J. P. (1998). "Bilateral testicular tumors: management and outcome in 21 patients." Cancer 83(3): 547-552.

de Gouveia Brazao, C. A., Pierik, F. H., Oosterhuis, J. W., Dohle, G. R., Looijenga, L. H. & Weber, R. F. (2004). "Bilateral testicular microlithiasis predicts the presence of the precursor of testicular germ cell tumors in subfertile men." J Urol 171(1): 158-160.

de Jong, J., Stoop, H., Dohle, G. R., Bangma, C. H., Kliffen, M., van Esser, J. W., van den Bent, M., Kros, J. M., Oosterhuis, J. W. & Looijenga, L. H. (2005). "Diagnostic value of OCT3/4 for pre-invasive and invasive testicular germ cell tumours." J Pathol 206(2): 242-249.

DeCastro, B. J., Peterson, A. C. & Costabile, R. A. (2008). "A 5-year followup study of asymptomatic men with testicular microlithiasis." J Urol 179(4): 1420-1423; discussion 1423.

Di Vizio, D., Cito, L., Boccia, A., Chieffi, P., Insabato, L., Pettinato, G., Motti, M. L., Schepis, F., D'Amico, W., Fabiani, F., Tavernise, B., Venuta, S., Fusco, A. & Viglietto, G. (2005). "Loss of the tumor suppressor gene PTEN marks the transition from intratubular germ cell neoplasias (ITGCN) to invasive germ cell tumors." Oncogene 24(11): 1882-1894.

Dieckmann, K. P., Heinemann, V., Frey, U. & Pichlmeier, U. (2005). "How harmful is contralateral testicular biopsy?--an analysis of serial imaging studies and a prospective evaluation of surgical complications." Eur Urol 48(4): 662-672.

Dieckmann, K. P., Kulejewski, M., Heinemann, V. & Loy, V. (2011). "Testicular biopsy for early cancer detection--objectives, technique and controversies." Int J Androl 34(4 Pt 2): e7-13.

Dieckmann, K. P., Kulejewski, M., Pichlmeier, U. & Loy, V. (2007). "Diagnosis of contralateral testicular intraepithelial neoplasia (TIN) in patients with testicular germ cell cancer: systematic two-site biopsies are more sensitive than a single random biopsy." Eur Urol 51(1): 175-183; discussion 183-175.

Dieckmann, K. P., Lauke, H., Michl, U., Winter, E. & Loy, V. (2002). "Testicular germ cell cancer despite previous local radiotherapy to the testis." Eur Urol 41(6): 643-649; discussion 649-650.

Dieckmann, K. P. & Loy, V. (1996). "Prevalence of contralateral testicular intraepithelial neoplasia in patients with testicular germ cell neoplasms." J Clin Oncol 14(12): 3126-3132.

Dieckmann, K. P. & Loy, V. (2003). "False-negative biopsies for the diagnosis of testicular intraepithelial neoplasia (TIN)--an update." Eur Urol 43(5): 516-521.

Dieckmann, K. P., Loy, V. & Buttner, P. (1993). "Prevalence of bilateral testicular germ cell tumours and early detection based on contralateral testicular intra-epithelial neoplasia." Br J Urol 71(3): 340-345.

Dieckmann, K. P. & Skakkebaek, N. E. (1999). "Carcinoma in situ of the testis: review of biological and clinical features." Int J Cancer 83(6): 815-822.

Dotsch, M., Brauers, A., Buttner, R., Nolte-Ernsting, C., Eble, M. J. & Jakse, G. (2000). "Malignant germ cell tumor of the contralateral testis after radiotherapy for testicular intraepithelial neoplasia." J Urol 164(2): 452-453.

Elzinga-Tinke, J. E., Sirre, M. E., Looijenga, L. H., van Casteren, N., Wildhagen, M. F. & Dohle, G. R. (2010). "The predictive value of testicular ultrasound abnormalities for carcinoma in situ of the testis in men at risk for testicular cancer." Int J Androl 33(4): 597-603.

Emerson, R. E. & Ulbright, T. M. (2010). "Intratubular germ cell neoplasia of the testis and its associated cancers: the use of novel biomarkers." Pathology 42(4): 344-355.

Fossa, S. D., Chen, J., Schonfeld, S. J., McGlynn, K. A., McMaster, M. L., Gail, M. H. & Travis, L. B. (2005). "Risk of contralateral testicular cancer: a population-based study of 29,515 U.S. men." J Natl Cancer Inst 97(14): 1056-1066.

Giwercman, A., Andrews, P. W., Jorgensen, N., Muller, J., Graem, N. & Skakkebaek, N. E. (1993a). "Immunohistochemical expression of embryonal marker TRA-1-60 in carcinoma in situ and germ cell tumors of the testis." Cancer 72(4): 1308-1314.

Giwercman, A., Bruun, E., Frimodt-Moller, C. & Skakkebaek, N. E. (1989). "Prevalence of carcinoma in situ and other histopathological abnormalities in testes of men with a history of cryptorchidism." J Urol 142(4): 998-1001; discussion 1001-1002.

Giwercman, A., Hopman, A. H., Ramaekers, F. C. & Skakkebaek, N. E. (1990a). "Carcinoma in situ of the testis. Detection of malignant germ cells in seminal fluid by means of in situ hybridization." Am J Pathol 136(3): 497-502.

Giwercman, A., Lindenberg, S., Kimber, S. J., Andersson, T., Muller, J. & Skakkebaek, N. E. (1990b). "Monoclonal antibody 43-9F as a sensitive immunohistochemical marker of carcinoma in situ of human testis." Cancer 65(5): 1135-1142.

Giwercman, A., Marks, A., Bailey, D., Baumal, R. & Skakkebaek, N. E. (1988a). "A monoclonal antibody as a marker for carcinoma in situ germ cells of the human adult testis." APMIS 96(8): 667-670.

Giwercman, A., Marks, A. & Skakkebaek, N. E. (1988b). "Carcinoma-in-situ germ-cells exfoliated from seminiferous epithelium into seminal fluid." Lancet 1(8584): 530.

Giwercman, A., Muller, J. & Skakkebaek, N. E. (1991a). "Prevalence of carcinoma in situ and other histopathological abnormalities in testes from 399 men who died suddenly and unexpectedly." J Urol 145(1): 77-80.

Giwercman, A., von der Maase, H., Berthelsen, J. G., Rorth, M., Bertelsen, A. & Skakkebaek, N. E. (1991b). "Localized irradiation of testes with carcinoma in situ: effects on Leydig cell function and eradication of malignant germ cells in 20 patients." J Clin Endocrinol Metab 73(3): 596-603.

Giwercman, A., von der Maase, H., Rorth, M. & Skakkebaek, N. E. (1993b). "Semen quality in testicular tumour and CIS in the contralateral testis." Lancet 341(8841): 384-385.

Gondos, B., Berthelsen, J. G. & Skakkebaek, N. E. (1983). "Intratubular germ cell neoplasia (carcinoma in situ): a preinvasive lesion of the testis." Ann Clin Lab Sci 13(3): 185-192.

Gondos, B. & Migliozzi, J. A. (1987). "Intratubular germ cell neoplasia." Semin Diagn Pathol 4(4): 292-303.

Grigor, K. M. & Rorth, M. (1993). "Should the contralateral testis be biopsied? Round table discussion." Eur Urol 23(1): 129-135.

Harland, S. J., Cook, P. A., Fossa, S. D., Horwich, A., Mead, G. M., Parkinson, M. C., Roberts, J. T. & Stenning, S. P. (1998). "Intratubular germ cell neoplasia of the contralateral testis in testicular cancer: defining a high risk group." J Urol 160(4): 1353-1357.

Harland, S. J., Cook, P. A., Fossa, S. D., Horwich, A., Parkinson, M. C., Roberts, J. T. & Stenning, S. P. (1993). "Risk factors for carcinoma in situ of the contralateral testis in patients with testicular cancer. An interim report." Eur Urol 23(1): 115-118; discussion 119.

Hart, A. H., Hartley, L., Parker, K., Ibrahim, M., Looijenga, L. H., Pauchnik, M., Chow, C. W. & Robb, L. (2005). "The pluripotency homeobox gene NANOG is expressed in human germ cell tumors." Cancer 104(10): 2092-2098.

Heidenreich, A. (2009). "Contralateral testicular biopsy in testis cancer: current concepts and controversies." BJU Int 104(9 Pt B): 1346-1350.

Heidenreich, A. & Moul, J. W. (2002). "Contralateral testicular biopsy procedure in patients with unilateral testis cancer: is it indicated?" Semin Urol Oncol 20(4): 234-238.

Heidenreich, A., Vorreuther, R., Neubauer, S., Zumbe, J. & Engelmann, U. H. (1997). "Paternity in patients with bilateral testicular germ cell tumors." Eur Urol 31(2): 246-248.

Heidenreich, A., Weissbach, L., Holtl, W., Albers, P., Kliesch, S., Kohrmann, K. U. & KP, D. I. (2001). "Organ sparing surgery for malignant germ cell tumor of the testis." J Urol 166(6): 2161-2165.

Hemminki, K. & Li, X. (2002). "Cancer risks in second-generation immigrants to Sweden." Int J Cancer 99(2): 229-237.

Hentrich, M., Weber, N., Bergsdorf, T., Liedl, B., Hartenstein, R. & Gerl, A. (2005). "Management and outcome of bilateral testicular germ cell tumors: Twenty-five year experience in Munich." Acta Oncol 44(6): 529-536.

Hoei-Hansen, C. E., Almstrup, K., Nielsen, J. E., Brask Sonne, S., Graem, N., Skakkebaek, N. E., Leffers, H. & Rajpert-De Meyts, E. (2005a). "Stem cell pluripotency factor NANOG is expressed in human fetal gonocytes, testicular carcinoma in situ and germ cell tumours." Histopathology 47(1): 48-56.

Hoei-Hansen, C. E., Nielsen, J. E., Almstrup, K., Hansen, M. A., Skakkebaek, N. E., Rajpert-DeMeyts, E. & Leffers, H. (2004a). "Identification of genes differentially expressed in testes containing carcinoma in situ." Mol Hum Reprod 10(6): 423-431.

Hoei-Hansen, C. E., Nielsen, J. E., Almstrup, K., Sonne, S. B., Graem, N., Skakkebaek, N. E., Leffers, H. & Rajpert-De Meyts, E. (2004b). "Transcription factor AP-2gamma is a developmentally regulated marker of testicular carcinoma in situ and germ cell tumors." Clin Cancer Res 10(24): 8521-8530.

Hoei-Hansen, C. E., Rajpert-De Meyts, E., Daugaard, G. & Skakkebaek, N. E. (2005b). "Carcinoma in situ testis, the progenitor of testicular germ cell tumours: a clinical review." Ann Oncol 16(6): 863-868.

Holm, M., Hoei-Hansen, C. E., Rajpert-De Meyts, E. & Skakkebaek, N. E. (2003). "Increased risk of carcinoma in situ in patients with testicular germ cell cancer with ultrasonic microlithiasis in the contralateral testicle." J Urol 170(4 Pt 1): 1163-1167.

Holstein, A. F. & Korner, F. (1974). "Light and electron microscopical analysis of cell types in human seminoma." Virchows Arch A Pathol Anat Histol 363(2): 97-112.

Holstein, A. F. & Lauke, H. (1996). "Histologic diagnostics of early testicular germ-cell tumor." Int J Urol 3(3): 165-172.

Holzbeierlein, J. M., Sogani, P. C. & Sheinfeld, J. (2003). "Histology and clinical outcomes in patients with bilateral testicular germ cell tumors: the Memorial Sloan Kettering Cancer Center experience 1950 to 2001." J Urol 169(6): 2122-2125.

Howlader, N., Noone, A. M., Krapcho, M., Neyman, N., Aminou, R., Waldron, W., Altekruse, S. F., Kosary, C. L., Ruhl, J., Tatalovich, Z., Cho, H., Mariotto, A., Eisner, M. P., Lewis, D. R., Chen, H. S., Feuer, E. J., Cronin, K. A. & Edwards, B. K. (2011). "SEER Cancer Statistics Review, 1975-2008." National Cancer Institute. Bethesda, MD.

Huyghe, E., Matsuda, T. & Thonneau, P. (2003). "Increasing incidence of testicular cancer worldwide: a review." J Urol 170(1): 5-11.

Huyghe, E., Muller, A., Mieusset, R., Bujan, L., Bachaud, J. M., Chevreau, C., Plante, P. & Thonneau, P. (2007). "Impact of diagnostic delay in testis cancer: results of a large population-based study." Eur Urol 52(6): 1710-1716.

Ikinger, U., Wurster, K., Terwey, B. & Mohring, K. (1982). "Microcalcifications in testicular malignancy: diagnostic tool in occult tumor?" Urology 19(5): 525-528.

Jacobsen, G. K., Henriksen, O. B. & von der Maase, H. (1981). "Carcinoma in situ of testicular tissue adjacent to malignant germ-cell tumors: a study of 105 cases." Cancer 47(11): 2660-2662.

Jacobsen, G. K. & Norgaard-Pedersen, B. (1984). "Placental alkaline phosphatase in testicular germ cell tumours and in carcinoma-in-situ of the testis. An immunohistochemical study." Acta Pathol Microbiol Immunol Scand A 92(5): 323-329.

Jones, T. D., MacLennan, G. T., Bonnin, J. M., Varsegi, M. F., Blair, J. E. & Cheng, L. (2006). "Screening for intratubular germ cell neoplasia of the testis using OCT4 immunohistochemistry." Am J Surg Pathol 30(11): 1427-1431.

Jones, T. D., Ulbright, T. M., Eble, J. N. & Cheng, L. (2004). "OCT4: A sensitive and specific biomarker for intratubular germ cell neoplasia of the testis." Clin Cancer Res 10(24): 8544-8547.

Jorgensen, N., Giwercman, A., Muller, J. & Skakkebaek, N. E. (1993). "Immunohistochemical markers of carcinoma in situ of the testis also expressed in normal infantile germ cells." Histopathology 22(4): 373-378.

Kleinschmidt, K., Dieckmann, K. P., Georgiew, A., Loy, V. & Weissbach, L. (2009). "Chemotherapy is of limited efficacy in the control of contralateral testicular intraepithelial neoplasia in patients with testicular germ cell cancer." Oncology 77(1): 33-39.

Kliesch, S., Thomaidis, T., Schutte, B., Puhse, G., Kater, B., Roth, S. & Bergmann, M. (2003). "Update on the diagnostic safety for detection of testicular intraepithelial neoplasia (TIN)." APMIS 111(1): 70-74; discussion 75.

Krabbe, S., Skakkebaek, N. E., Berthelsen, J. G., Eyben, F. V., Volsted, P., Mauritzen, K., Eldrup, J. & Nielsen, A. H. (1979). "High incidence of undetected neoplasia in maldescended testes." Lancet 1(8124): 999-1000.

Lacerda, H. M., Akre, O., Merletti, F. & Richiardi, L. (2009). "Time trends in the incidence of testicular cancer in childhood and young adulthood." Cancer Epidemiol Biomarkers Prev 18(7): 2042-2045.

Lauke, H. (1997). "Rapid method to detect CIS-cells." Adv Exp Med Biol 424: 69-70.

Lenz, S., Skakkebaek, N. E. & Hertel, N. T. (1996). "Abnormal ultrasonic pattern in contralateral testes in patients with unilateral testicular cancer." World J Urol 14 Suppl 1: S55-58.

Linke, J., Loy, V. & Dieckmann, K. P. (2005). "Prevalence of testicular intraepithelial neoplasia in healthy males." J Urol 173(5): 1577-1579.

Looijenga, L. H., Zafarana, G., Grygalewicz, B., Summersgill, B., Debiec-Rychter, M., Veltman, J., Schoenmakers, E. F., Rodriguez, S., Jafer, O., Clark, J., van Kessel, A. G., Shipley, J., van Gurp, R. J., Gillis, A. J. & Oosterhuis, J. W. (2003). "Role of gain of 12p in germ cell tumour development." APMIS 111(1): 161-171; discussion 172-163.

Loy, V., Wigand, I. & Dieckmann, K. P. (1990). "Incidence and distribution of carcinoma in situ in testes removed for germ cell tumour: possible inadequacy of random testicular biopsy in detecting the condition." Histopathology 16(2): 198-200.

Manivel, J. C., Jessurun, J., Wick, M. R. & Dehner, L. P. (1987). "Placental alkaline phosphatase immunoreactivity in testicular germ-cell neoplasms." Am J Surg Pathol 11(1): 21-29.

Manning, M., Junemann, K. P. & Alken, P. (1998). "Decrease in testosterone blood concentrations after testicular sperm extraction for intracytoplasmic sperm injection in azoospermic men." Lancet 352(9121): 37.

Mark, G. J. & Hedinger, C. (1965). "Changes in remaining tumor-free testicular tissue in cases of seminoma and teratoma." Virchows Arch Pathol Anat Physiol Klin Med 340(1): 84-92.

Moller, H. (1989). "Decreased testicular cancer risk in men born in wartime." J Natl Cancer Inst 81(21): 1668-1669.

Moller, H. (1993). "Clues to the aetiology of testicular germ cell tumours from descriptive epidemiology." Eur Urol 23(1): 8-13; discussion 14-15.

Mortensen, M. S., Gundgaard, M. G. & Daugaard, G. (2011). "Treatment options for carcinoma in situ testis." Int J Androl 34(4 Pt 2): e32-36.

Muller, J., Skakkebaek, N. E., Nielsen, O. H. & Graem, N. (1984). "Cryptorchidism and testis cancer. Atypical infantile germ cells followed by carcinoma in situ and invasive carcinoma in adulthood." Cancer 54(4): 629-634.

Myrup, C., Westergaard, T., Schnack, T., Oudin, A., Ritz, C., Wohlfahrt, J. & Melbye, M. (2008). "Testicular cancer risk in first- and second-generation immigrants to Denmark." J Natl Cancer Inst 100(1): 41-47.

Myrup, C., Wohlfahrt, J., Oudin, A., Schnack, T. & Melbye, M. (2010). "Risk of testicular cancer according to birthplace and birth cohort in Denmark." Int J Cancer 126(1): 217-223.

Olesen, I. A., Hoei-Hansen, C. E., Skakkebaek, N. E., Petersen, J. H., Rajpert-De Meyts, E. & Jorgensen, N. (2007). "Testicular carcinoma in situ in subfertile Danish men." Int J Androl 30(4): 406-411; discussion 412.

Pamenter, B., De Bono, J. S., Brown, I. L., Nandini, M., Kaye, S. B., Russell, J. M., Yates, A. J. & Kirk, D. (2003). "Bilateral testicular cancer: a preventable problem? Experience from a large cancer centre." BJU Int 92(1): 43-46.

Petersen, P. M., Giwercman, A., Daugaard, G., Rorth, M., Petersen, J. H., Skakkeaek, N. E., Hansen, S. W. & von der Maase, H. (2002). "Effect of graded testicular doses of radiotherapy in patients treated for carcinoma-in-situ in the testis." J Clin Oncol 20(6): 1537-1543.

Petersen, P. M., Giwercman, A., Hansen, S. W., Berthelsen, J. G., Daugaard, G., Rorth, M. & Skakkebaek, N. E. (1999). "Impaired testicular function in patients with carcinoma-in-situ of the testis." J Clin Oncol 17(1): 173-179.

Ploen, L. & Setchell, B. P. (1992). "Blood-testis barriers revisited. A homage to Lennart Nicander." Int J Androl 15(1): 1-4.

Prym, C. & Lauke, H. (1994). "Carcinoma-in situ of the human testis: tumour cells are distributed focally in the seminiferous tubules." Andrologia 26(4): 231-234.

Pryor, J. P., Cameron, K. M., Chilton, C. P., Ford, T. F., Parkinson, M. C., Sinokrot, J. & Westwood, C. A. (1983). "Carcinoma in situ in testicular biopsies from men presenting with infertility." Br J Urol 55(6): 780-784.

Rajpert-De Meyts, E. (2006). "Developmental model for the pathogenesis of testicular carcinoma in situ: genetic and environmental aspects." Hum Reprod Update 12(3): 303-323.

Rajpert-De Meyts, E. & Skakkebaek, N. E. (1994). "Expression of the c-kit protein product in carcinoma-in-situ and invasive testicular germ cell tumours." Int J Androl 17(2): 85-92.

Sanli, O., Kadioglu, A., Atar, M., Acar, O. & Nane, I. (2008). "Grading of classical testicular microlithiasis has no effect on the prevalence of associated testicular tumors." Urol Int 80(3): 310-316.

Sedlmayer, F., Holtl, W., Kozak, W., Hawliczek, R., Gebhart, F., Gerber, E., Joos, H., Albrecht, W., Pummer, K. & Kogelnik, H. D. (2001). "Radiotherapy of testicular intraepithelial neoplasia (TIN): a novel treatment regimen for a rare disease." Int J Radiat Oncol Biol Phys 50(4): 909-913.

Skakkebaek, N. E. (1972). "Possible carcinoma-in-situ of the testis." Lancet 2(7776): 516-517.

Skakkebaek, N. E. (1975). "Atypical germ cells in the adjacent "normal" tissue of testicular tumours." Acta Pathol Microbiol Scand A 83(1): 127-130.

Skakkebaek, N. E. (1978). "Carcinoma in situ of the testis: frequency and relationship to invasive germ cell tumours in infertile men." Histopathology 2(3): 157-170.

Skakkebaek, N. E. (1979). "Carcinoma-in-situ of testis in testicular feminization syndrome." Acta Pathol Microbiol Scand A 87(1): 87-89.

Skakkebaek, N. E., Berthelsen, J. G., Giwercman, A. & Muller, J. (1987). "Carcinoma-in-situ of the testis: possible origin from gonocytes and precursor of all types of germ cell tumours except spermatocytoma." Int J Androl 10(1): 19-28.

Slowikowska-Hilczer, J., Szarras-Czapnik, M. & Kula, K. (2001). "Testicular pathology in 46,XY dysgenetic male pseudohermaphroditism: an approach to pathogenesis of testis cancer." J Androl 22(5): 781-792.

Sonne, S. B., Almstrup, K., Dalgaard, M., Juncker, A. S., Edsgard, D., Ruban, L., Harrison, N. J., Schwager, C., Abdollahi, A., Huber, P. E., Brunak, S., Gjerdrum, L. M., Moore, H. D., Andrews, P. W., Skakkebaek, N. E., Rajpert-De Meyts, E. & Leffers, H. (2009). "Analysis of gene expression profiles of microdissected cell populations indicates that testicular carcinoma in situ is an arrested gonocyte." Cancer Res 69(12): 5241-5250.

Souchon, R., Gertenbach, U., Dieckmann, K. P., Hahn, E., Ruwe, M., Stambolis, C., Loy, V. & Classen, J. (2006). "Contralateral testicular cancer in spite of TIN-negative double biopsies and interval cisplatin chemotherapy." Strahlenther Onkol 182(5): 289-292.

Summersgill, B., Osin, P., Lu, Y. J., Huddart, R. & Shipley, J. (2001). "Chromosomal imbalances associated with carcinoma in situ and associated testicular germ cell tumours of adolescents and adults." Br J Cancer 85(2): 213-220.

Tan, I. B., Ang, K. K., Ching, B. C., Mohan, C., Toh, C. K. & Tan, M. H. (2010). "Testicular microlithiasis predicts concurrent testicular germ cell tumors and intratubular germ cell neoplasia of unclassified type in adults: a meta-analysis and systematic review." Cancer 116(19): 4520-4532.

van Casteren, N. J., de Jong, J., Stoop, H., Steyerberg, E. W., de Bekker-Grob, E. W., Dohle, G. R., Oosterhuis, J. W. & Looijenga, L. H. (2009). "Evaluation of testicular biopsies for carcinoma in situ: immunohistochemistry is mandatory." Int J Androl 32(6): 666-674.

von der Maase, H., Berthelsen, J. G., Jacobsen, G. K., Hald, T., Rorth, M., Christophersen, I. S., Sorensen, B. L., Walbom-Jorgensen, S. & Skakkebaek, N. E. (1985). "Carcinoma-in-situ of testis eradicated by chemotherapy." Lancet 1(8420): 98.

von der Maase, H., Meinecke, B. & Skakkebaek, N. E. (1988). "Residual carcinoma-in-situ of contralateral testis after chemotherapy." Lancet 1(8583): 477-478.

von der Maase, H., Rorth, M., Walbom-Jorgensen, S., Sorensen, B. L., Christophersen, I. S., Hald, T., Jacobsen, G. K., Berthelsen, J. G. & Skakkebaek, N. E. (1986). "Carcinoma in situ of contralateral testis in patients with testicular germ cell cancer: study of 27 cases in 500 patients." Br Med J (Clin Res Ed) 293(6559): 1398-1401.

von Eckardstein, S., Tsakmakidis, G., Kamischke, A., Rolf, C. & Nieschlag, E. (2001). "Sonographic testicular microlithiasis as an indicator of premalignant conditions in normal and infertile men." J Androl 22(5): 818-824.

Walsh, T. J., Croughan, M. S., Schembri, M., Chan, J. M. & Turek, P. J. (2009). "Increased risk of testicular germ cell cancer among infertile men." Arch Intern Med 169(4): 351-356.

Wood, H. M. & Elder, J. S. (2009). "Cryptorchidism and testicular cancer: separating fact from fiction." J Urol 181(2): 452-461.

2

Management of Nonseminomatous Germ Cell Tumor of the Testis

Paul H. Johnston and Stephen D.W. Beck
Indiana University,
USA

1. Introduction

1.1 Management options for clinical stage I non-seminomatous germ cell tumor of the testis

1.1.1 Introduction to clinical stage I disease

About 5-7/100,000 men are diagnosed with testis cancer annually. A large proportion of these are pathologically classified as non-seminomatous germ cell tumor (NSGCT). The majority of NSGCT patients present with clinical stage (CS) I disease, which is characterized by a germ cell tumor confined to the testis, a negative metastatic work-up which includes a chest X-ray (CXR), computed tomography scan of the abdomen and pelvis (CT A&P), and negative serum tumor markers (STM) post-orchiectomy. Patients who present with CS I testis cancer have a 30 percent chance of harboring occult metastatic disease post-orchiectomy, and thus controversy exists as to what represents the best treatment strategy following radical orchiectomy. Currently, there are 3 treatment strategies available for patients with CS I testis cancer, each one associated with a 99% cure rate: surveillance, adjuvant chemotherapy, and primary retroperitoneal lymph node dissection (RPLND).

1.2 Risk stratification for stage I disease

The ability to risk classify CSI patients to "high risk" of harboring micrometastatic disease and "low risk" of having micrometastatic disease would aid in tailoring therapy. Those patients identified as "high risk" could more preferentially be treated with primary RPLND or adjuvant chemotherapy, as they would have a greater risk of relapse on surveillance. Conversely, "low risk" patients may be managed with surveillance as they would have a greater likelihood of being cured with orchiectomy alone and thus overtreated with primary RPLND or adjuvant chemotherapy.

Several key studies have been published identifying pathologic factors predictive of metastatic disease in these patients. In 1987, a retrospective MRC trial identified four important negative prognostic indicators: presence of embryonal carcinoma, absence of yolk sac tumor, vascular invasion of the primary tumor, and lymphatic invasion of the primary tumor. (Freedman et al., 1987) These risk factors were then evaluated prospectively, revealing the presence of 3 or more risk factors as predictive of recurrence in approximately

50% of patients, and the presence of 2 or less risk factors as predictive of micrometastatic disease in about 20% of patients. Notably, vascular invasion of the primary tumor was most predictive. (Read et al., 1992) More recently, Vergouwe et al. reviewed 23 publications assessing predictors of occult metastases. (Vergouwe, Steyerberg, Eijkemans, Albers, & Habbema, 2003) Of the 2,587 total patients involved, 759 (29.3%) patients had occult metastasis. Pooled univariate odds ratios identified that lymphovascular invasion of the primary tumor, embryonal carcinoma component representing >50% of tumor, advanced pathologic stage (T2-4 versus T1), and monoclonal antibody MIB-1 staining greater than 70% of the tumor as the strongest predictors of occult metastases. Though somewhat variable, high risk groups, with the presence of either or both lymphovascular invasion and an embryonal dominant primary, carried a recurrence rate of approximately 50%. In patients without either pathologic variable, a recurrence rate of less than 20% was observed.

At best, with current risk classification, 50% of the "high risk" group harbor micrometastatic disease and 50% are cured by orchiectomy alone. Thus any therapy beyond orchiectomy for the "high risk" group overtreats 50% of patients, who are never destined to relapse. As such, risk classification is less than ideal in determining treatment. Future research aims to improve the prognostic ability of risk classification.

1.3 Surveillance for clinical stage I disease

1.3.1 Clinical outcomes of surveillance

The primary rationale for surveillance as a therapeutic modality is: 1) it avoids any further therapy in the 70% patients who do not harbor micrometastatic disease and who were cured by orchiectomy alone, and 2) those 30% of patients that relapse are curable with chemotherapy and/or surgery. To achieve a high cure rate, all patients on surveillance must be adherent to a strict follow-up schedule to identify those destined to relapse.

While surveillance avoids therapy in the large proportion of patients who are not destined to recur, there remains a burden of therapy for those that do. Some surveillance patients relapsing in the retroperitoneum with normal serum tumor markers may be candidates for primary RPLND. The remainder will require 3 courses of chemotherapy, and approximately a quarter of these will require surgery following chemotherapy. In the single center surveillance series of testis cancer patients from Toronto, at a median follow up of 6.3 years, 104 of 371 (28%) patients relapsed on surveillance. (Kakiashvili, Zuniga, & Jewett, 2009) Of the 104 patients that recurred, the burden of therapy included chemotherapy alone in 31, surgery alone in 31, and a combination of chemotherapy, surgery and radiation in the remaining 42 patients. Similar results were seen in a cohort of 223 patients from British Columbia and Oregon, where 26% relapsed on surveillance. (Kollmannsberger et al., 2010) No deaths were observed among those who recurred, although 20% of those who relapsed (8% of the original cohort) required post-chemotherapy retroperitoneal lymph node dissection (PC RPLND) in addition to chemotherapy.

Despite those recurrences, the overall survival for patients on surveillance equals that of primary RPLND or adjuvant chemotherapy. In a pooled analysis of 3424 patients on surveillance in series that reported death, a 98.6% disease specific survival was demonstrated. (Groll, Warde, & Jewett, 2007)

1.3.2 Follow up for surveillance

While some patients on surveillance will bear the burden of therapy upon relapse, all patients on surveillance bear the burden of compliance. Studies indicate that up to a third of patients miss at least one clinic visit. (Divrik, Akdogan, Ozen, & Zorlu, 2006; Meinke, Estes, & Ernst, 1979) A recent evaluation of compliance of CS I patients at the University of Calgary showed extremely poor compliance with scheduled follow up. (Hao et al., 1998) In this study, compliance with clinic visits and tumor markers was only 61% during the first year and 35% in year 2. Furthermore, compliance with scheduled CT scans was only 25% in year 1 and 12% in year 2. The only two deaths in 76 total patients were in individuals who were non-compliant with follow up. There is concern that non-compliance may translate into a decrease in disease specific survival. (Colls et al., 1999; Gels et al., 1995; Kakehi, Kamoto, Kawakita, & Ogawa, 2002; Raghavan et al., 1988) Nevertheless, the true impact of non-compliance on survival is unknown. A national surveillance study in New Zealand failed to correlate non-compliance with compromise in cure. (Colls, et al., 1999)

In addition to the risk of poor compliance, some patients on a surveillance protocol will experience anxiety due to the possibility of relapse. Although such anxiety is difficult to quantify, it is understandable that for some patient personalities, active therapy by way of primary RPLND or chemotherapy would be more desirable.

The burden of compliance involves more than anxiety or clinic attendance. Compliance with scheduled imaging studies will result in increased radiation exposure, and this exposure carries a slightly increased risk of secondary malignancy in this young population. (Brenner & Hall, 2007) Given higher relapse rates in the first 2 years of surveillance, (Groll, et al., 2007) more intensive follow-up is required in this time period using a combination of physical exam, CXR, STM, and CT A&P. In an effort to minimize radiation exposure, a randomized trial evaluated CT A&P at 3 and 12 months versus 3, 6, 9, 12, and 24 months and found no detection benefit in more frequent imaging. This study involved 414 patients with a median follow-up of 40 months, though only 10% of the patients were considered high risk based on vascular invasion. (Rustin et al., 2007) A popular follow-up schedule is that of the Toronto group, which is of moderate frequency compared to the aforementioned schedules, and is outlined in Table 1.

	Month 2	Month 4	Month 6	Month 8	Month 10	Month 12
Year 1	STM,CXR	STM,CXR,CT A&P	STM, CXR	STM,CXR,CT A&P	STM, CXR	STM,CXR,CT A&P
Year 2	STM,CXR	STM,CXR,CT A&P	STM, CXR	STM,CXR,CT A&P	STM, CXR	STM,CXR,CT A&P
Year 3		STM,CXR		STM,CXR		STM,CXR
Year 4			STM,CXR			STM,CXR
Year 5						STM,CXR

Table 1. Toronto CS I NSGCT Surveillance Schedule

In addition to compliance issues, surveillance protocols also affect fertility rates, which approach 65% during surveillance, but decreases to 20% for surveillance patients that recur. (Herr, Bar-Chama, O'Sullivan, & Sogani, 1998).

1.3.3 Summary: Surveillance for clinical stage I disease

Surveillance offers an equal cure rate to either primary RPLND or adjuvant chemotherapy, and does so while avoiding further therapy in 70% of patients. Therefore, it is arguably the treatment option of choice in patients without significant pathologic risk factors for occult retroperitoneal metastases, who are willing to undergo serial imaging and intense follow-up. However, patients who choose surveillance must be aware of the importance of adherence to their follow-up schedule, and the fact that 30% of patients will require chemotherapy at relapse. As a result, patients strongly averse to chemotherapy may not wish to choose a surveillance protocol, favoring primary RPLND instead.

1.4 Adjuvant chemotherapy for clinical stage I disease

1.4.1 Clinical outcomes of adjuvant chemotherapy

The rationale for chemotherapy in CS I NSGCT is that it virtually eliminates the risk of recurrence, with an incidence rate much lower than that observed with either primary RPLND or surveillance. Recurrence rates were reported by the Spanish Germ Cell Group involving 231 high risk patients who received two courses of bleomycin, etoposide, and cisplatinum (BEP). (Maroto et al., 2005) Two patients (0.9%) relapsed and both are disease free after salvage therapy. Long-term follow up extending 10 years has confirmed the low relapse rates associated with adjuvant chemotherapy. (Chevreau et al., 2004; Westermann et al., 2008) Similarly low recurrence rates have been reported in other series also using 2 courses of BEP, (Cullen et al., 1996; Oliver, Raja, Ong, & Gallagher, 1992) allowing clinicians to draw the conclusion that there is little doubt on the efficacy of chemotherapy in preventing recurrence and achieving cure rates similar to surveillance or RPLND strategies for CS I NSGCT patients.

1.4.2 Morbidity of adjuvant chemotherapy

While the recurrence rates following 2 cycles of adjuvant BEP are impressively low, all patients, including the 70% who did not require this additional therapy, are subjected to the burden of systemic chemotherapy. Given the young age of most testis cancer patients, a lifetime remains to accrue complications secondary to this treatment choice. Specifically, the Royal Marsden Hospital reported a 2-fold greater risk of developing cardiovascular disease in testis cancer patients treated with chemotherapy and radiation. (Huddart et al., 2003) Others have reported that cured patients treated with cisplatin-based chemotherapy have a higher prevalence of hypertension and an excessive weight gain compared with patients treated with other modalities, and compared to controls. (Sagstuen et al., 2005) A recent report evaluated the long-term toxicity of cisplatin-based chemotherapy in 1409 men at a median follow-up of 10.7 years. (Brydoy et al., 2009) All chemotherapy groups had statistically higher odds of toxicity than men who did not receive chemotherapy, and that toxicity most commonly included Raynaud-like phenomena in 39%, paresthesias in the hands or feet in 29%, hearing impairment in 21% and tinnitus in 22%. Finally, it is worth noting that fertility rates during chemotherapy will drop substantially, recovering to approximately an 85% conception rate for couples desiring children, with a mean of 3 years of follow up. (Huyghe et al., 2004)

Bearing these concerning morbidity rates in mind, efforts have been made to decrease the toxicity of chemotherapy regimens by decreasing dose rates. Investigators have attempted to decrease the exposure to chemotherapy by treating clinical stage I patients with a single cycle of BEP. The Swiss Group for Clinical Cancer Research reported outcomes of high risk stage I patients receiving a single course of BEP in the adjuvant setting. (Westermann, et al., 2008) Data from 40 of the 44 patients were analyzed. Thirty-five showed no evidence of disease during a median follow up of 99 months. One patient developed pulmonary metastases after 13 months and died of pneumonia. Two patients developed contralateral testis cancer, subsequently received three cycles of BEP, and were relapse free for 4 and 92 months, respectively, thereafter. Two final patients were free of disease at 10 and 31 months when lost to follow-up. Also utilizing one course of BEP, the German Testicular Cancer Study Group has reported a 2-year disease free survival of 99.5% after a median follow up of 4.7 years, with just 2 recurrences observed in the intention-to-treat population. (Albers et al., 2008)

1.4.3 Follow up for adjuvant chemotherapy

During chemotherapy, serum markers are monitored prior to each cycle. Upon completion of 2 cycles of BEP, patient follow-up need be tailored based upon individual patient outcomes, and will include periodic physical examination, serum markers, and imaging of the chest, abdomen, and pelvis. (L. Wood et al., 2010)

1.4.4 Summary: Adjuvant chemotherapy for clinical stage I disease

To summarize chemotherapy as a treatment option, its greatest advantage lies in its recurrence rate of less than 2%. However, it subjects all patients, including the 70% never destined to recur, to the short and long term complications of systemic chemotherapy. While recent data suggest that one cycle of BEP may be adequate to achieve acceptably low recurrence rates, the standard of care continues to be two cycles of BEP, and the attendant morbidities of this therapeutic choice must be borne in mind.

1.5 Primary RPLND for clinical stage I disease

1.5.1 Clinical outcomes of primary RPLND – pathologic stage I disease

Testis cancer is unique among urologic cancers in that surgery (RPLND) can cure patients that have metastatic disease. Of CS I patients choosing primary RPLND, 70% will have no metastatic disease in their retroperitoneum, and are classified as pathologic stage I. Despite negative lymph nodes, 10% will relapse, and thus these patients still require follow-up. The remaining 30% with occult cancer identified in the lymph nodes are classified as pathologic stage II. For patients with pathologic stage II disease, surgery alone is curative in approximately 70%, and those 30% that relapse are cured with chemotherapy. Irrespective of pathologic stage, 99% patients who choose primary RPLND will ultimately be cured of their disease. (Donohue, Thornhill, Foster, Rowland, & Bihrle, 1993b)

1.5.2 Clinical outcomes of primary RPLND – low volume pathologic stage II disease

Management options for pathologic stage II disease include observation or adjuvant chemotherapy, as both have equal survival. This is based on a randomized trial of pathologic stage II patients which compared adjuvant chemotherapy to close observation (with chemotherapy for recurrence). (Williams, et al., 1987) Analysis revealed no difference in survival (95%) between the two treatment arms at a median follow-up of 4 years.

Outcomes for patients with low volume pathologic stage II disease who choose observation are well described in the literature. Pathologic stage II disease was identified in 112 of 464 patients undergoing primary RPLND at Indiana for what was originally staged as clinical stage I disease, from 1965 to 1989. (Donohue, Thornhill, Foster, Rowland, & Bihrle, 1993c) Sixty-six percent of those patients with pathologic stage II disease were cured by RPLND alone. Memorial Sloan Kettering reported an 81% four-year progression free probability for pathologic stage II patients who did not receive adjuvant chemotherapy following a full, bilateral RPLND with less than a 2cm retroperitoneal mass. (Stephenson et al., 2005) Similar results were obtained in a series from Indiana University which included 118 RPLND patients with pathologic stage II disease, who did not receive adjuvant chemotherapy, and were followed for a minimum of 2 years. The 5 year disease free survival for this cohort was 68%. (S. D. Beck, Foster, Bihrle, Cheng, & Donohue, 2005; S. D. Beck et al., 2005)

Thus, 70% of patients with pathologic stage II disease are cured with RPLND alone, and those 30% that do relapse remain curable with 3 courses of chemotherapy. An alternative approach in managing pathologic stage II disease is 2 courses of adjuvant chemotherapy. While this approach reduces recurrence rates to less than 2%, (Behnia, Foster, Einhorn, Donohue, & Nichols, 2000; Culine et al., 1996; Gerl, Clemm, Kohl, & al., 1994; Kennedy, Torkelson, & Fraley, 1994; Kondagunta et al., 2004; Vugrin, Whitmore, Herr, Sogani, & Golbey, 1982; Weissbach & Hartlapp, 1991; Williams et al., 1987) it subjects all patients to chemotherapy, including the 70% who were cured by surgery alone. (Donohue, Thornhill, Foster, Rowland, & Bihrle, 1993a, 1995a; Richie & Kantoff, 1991)

Similar to risk stratification in CS I disease, efforts have been made to identify risk factors predictive of relapse for pathologic stage II disease after RPLND. Knowledge of such risk factors would allow "high risk" patients to receive adjuvant chemotherapy, and "low risk" patients to be observed. To date, no pathologic or clinical variable has been identified to predict relapse. (S. D. Beck, et al., 2007) (S. D. Beck, R. S. Foster, R. Bihrle, L. Cheng, & J. P. Donohue, 2005) (S. D. Beck, R. S. Foster, R. Bihrle, L. Cheng, T. M. Ulbright, et al., 2005) (Rabbani et al., 2001) (Richie & Kantoff, 1991)

1.5.3 Primary RPLND technique

The traditional full bilateral suprahilar RPLND involved removal of all lymphatic tissue from the suprahilar areas to the bifurcation of the common iliac arteries, from ureter to contralateral ureter. This was, by intent, a radical procedure, because chemotherapeutic rescue was not available when full bilateral RPLND was initially developed. All sympathetic efferent fibers were sacrificed, and lymphatic tissue was removed en bloc. Therefore, these patients suffered from anejaculation post-operatively.

Since the original extent of dissection was developed, it has been discovered, through the advent of CT scanning, and with the aid of meticulous anatomic mapping studies, that patients with clinical stage I disease may be treated with a much more limited dissection in the retroperitoneum, ipsilateral to the affected testis. Specifically, patients with low-volume retroperitoneal tumor from a left sided primary characteristically had metastases localized to the upper left periaortic zone, and patients with low-volume disease from a right-sided primary were found to have metastases to the interaortocaval or precaval zones. These facts led investigators to modify the traditional full bilateral RPLND further and limit the dissection to the left- and right-sided templates, as depicted in Figures 1 and 2.

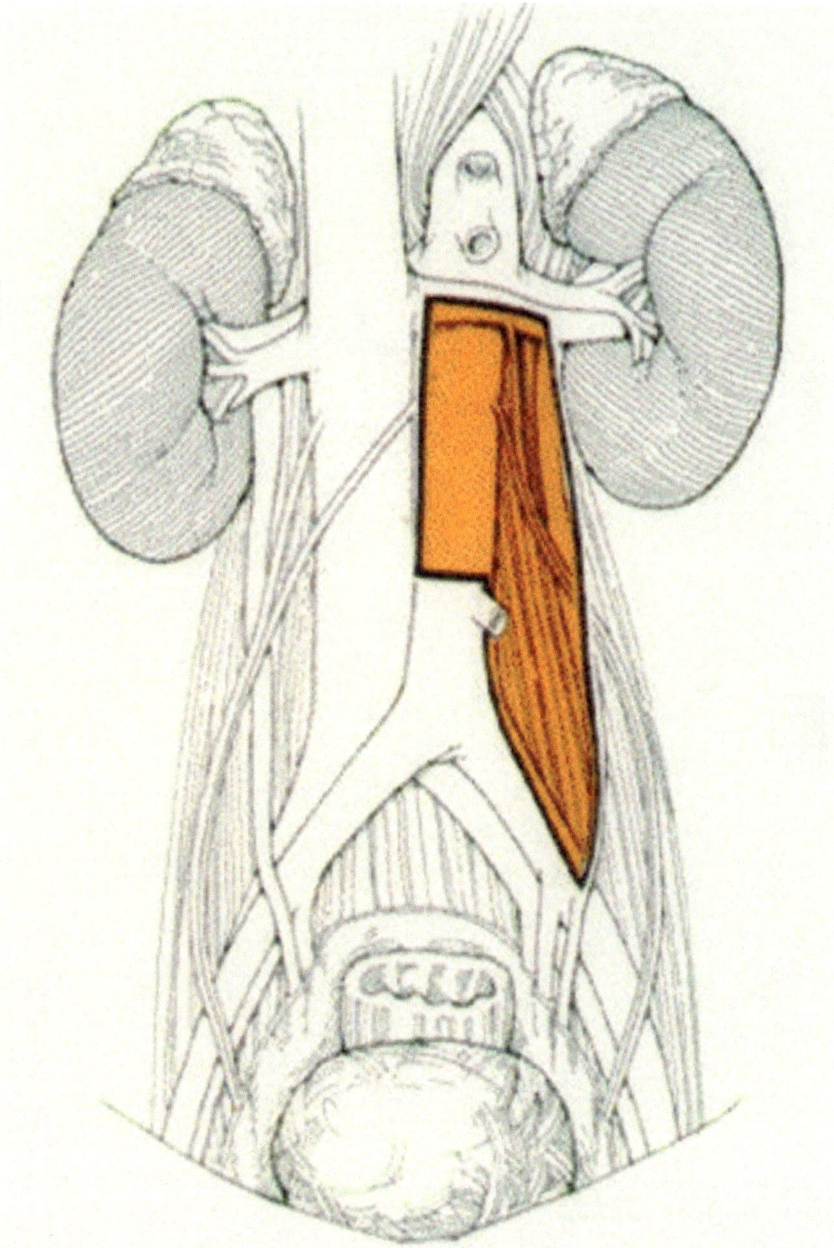

Fig. 1. Left-sided RPLND Template. Artist's rendering of the retroperitoneum. Orange area depicts area of surgical dissection.

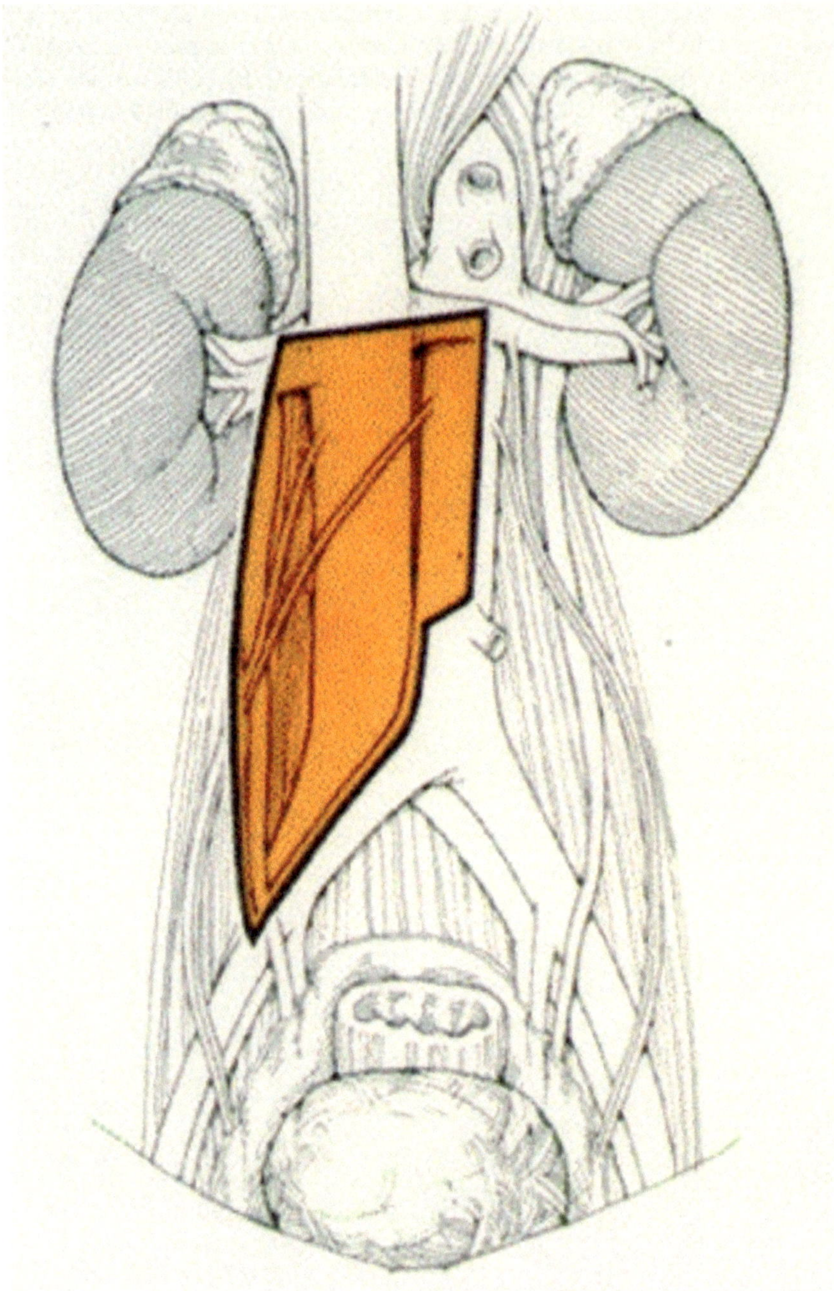

Fig. 2. Right-sided RPLND Template. Artist's rendering of the retroperitoneum. Orange area depicts area of surgical dissection.

With these templates, right and left sided dissection would remove lymphatic tissue at high risk of harboring metastatic disease, but preserve other retroperitoneal lymphatic tissue at low risk of containing metastasis. The advantages of limiting the dissection in patients with low volume disease were shorter operative times, and shorter postoperative ileus. Additionally, and most importantly, these templates saved contralateral retroperitoneal efferent sympathetic fibers, thereby preserving emission and ejaculation in roughly 50% to 70% of patients.

The most recent modification in technique for RPLND for low-stage disease is the nerve-sparing dissection, in which efferent sympathetic fibers are prospectively identified and dissected, and modified lymphadenectomy is then performed. This advancement in technique preserves the staging and therapeutic aspect of RPLND, while additionally improving upon ejaculation preservation rates. In Figure 3, the right-sided post-synaptic sympathetic nerves are enveloped by vessel loops, and are seen exiting the sympathetic chain from underneath an anteriorly retracted inferior vena cava (IVC).

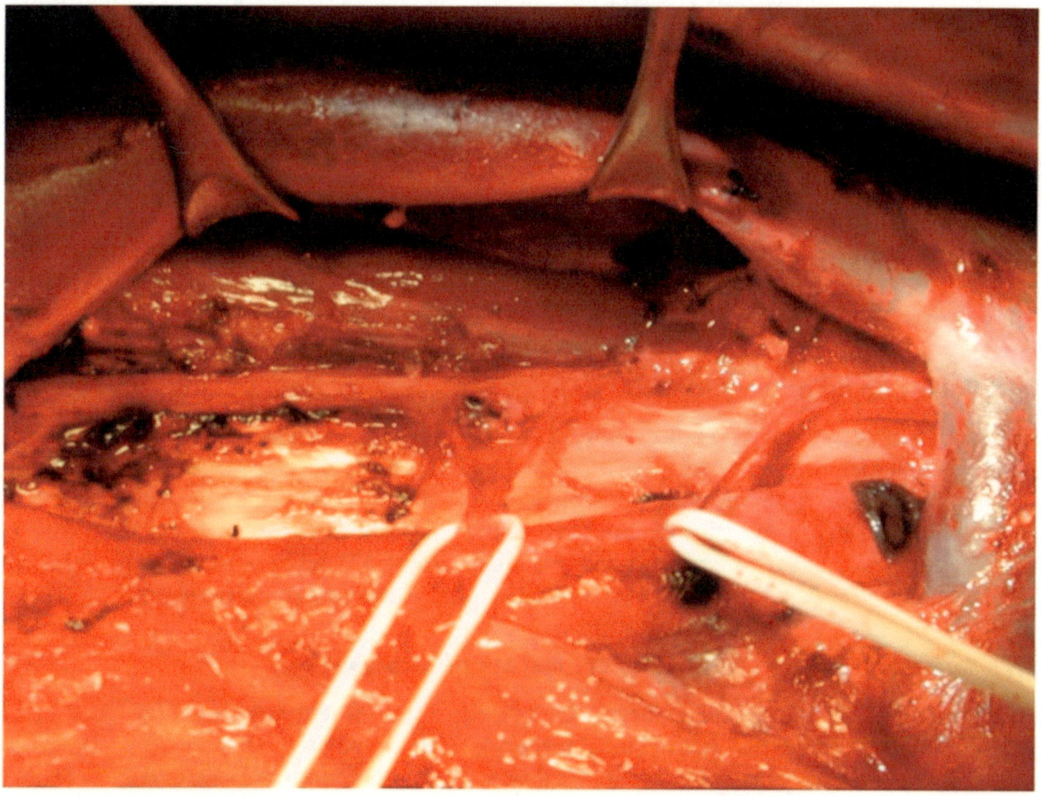

Fig. 3. Nerve-Sparing RPLND Technique. A photograph of the retroperitoneum during RPLND. The post-synaptic sympathetic nerves are encircled by white vessel loops for better visualization. Following the course of these nerves proximally, they can be seen joining the right sympathetic chain, which travels parallel and posterior to the inferior vena cava. The inferior vena cava is retracted anteriorly with vein retractors, to allow better visualization of the sympathetic chain.

A laparoscopic technique has been developed in an effort to further diminish primary RPLND's already favorable morbidity profile. It remains unknown as to whether or not the laparoscopic technique offers a morbidity benefit compared to the open technique. (Abdel-Aziz et al., 2006; Albqami & Janetschek, 2005; Janetschek, Hobisch, Holtl, & Bartsch, 1996;

Kenney & Tuerk, 2008) Furthermore, the vast majority of laparoscopic primary RPLND patients receive adjuvant chemotherapy following surgery, thus the therapeutic benefit of laparoscopic RPLND alone also remains unknown. (Rassweiler, Scheitlin, Heidenreich, Laguna, & Janetschek, 2008)

1.5.4 Morbidity of primary RPLND

Although primary RPLND as a treatment strategy offers excellent cure rates, it nonetheless subjects 70% of patients to unnecessary surgery. Fortunately, the morbidity of a primary RPLND is essentially that of a laparotomy. (Foster et al., 1994; Heidenreich et al., 2003; Jewett, 1990) A review of the experience at Indiana University showed that the only significant long-term morbidity is an approximate 1% chance of postoperative small bowel obstruction due to adhesions. (Baniel, Foster, Rowland, Bihrle, & Donohue, 1994) The same institution recently reviewed 75 consecutive primary retroperitoneal lymph node dissections. (S.D.W. Beck, Peterson, Foster, Bihrle, & Donohue, 2006) In this population the mean operative time was 132 minutes, mean blood loss was 207 cc. Nasogastric tubes are not routinely used in either primary or post chemotherapy surgery, and in this series only 2 patients had NG tubes. The mean hospital stay was 2.8 days (range: 2-4). With nerve-sparing technique, 99% maintain antegrade ejaculation, and a 75% fertility rate is observed. (S. D. Beck, Bey, Bihrle, & Foster, 2010; Foster et al., 1994) (S. D. Beck, Bey, Bihrle, & Foster, 2010; Foster, et al., 1994) This compares favorably to fertility rates for surveillance, and is roughly equivalent to fertility rates seen with chemotherapy.

1.5.5 Follow up for primary RPLND

Irrespective of pathologic stage at primary RPLND, the risk of relapse in the retroperitoneum is exceedingly low, with most relapses identified by chest X-ray and/or serum tumor markers. As such abdominal imaging with CT scan is not routinely used and follow-up consists of periodic chest X-ray, serum tumor markers, and physical examination. Given the rarity of relapse more than 2 years after remission, especially in the RPLND population, (Baniel et al., 1995) further follow-up accordingly becomes less rigorous in subsequent years.

1.5.6 Summary: Primary RPLND for clinical stage I disease

Though RPLND subjects all patients to a laparotomy (including the 70% that were pathologic stage I and did not require surgery), with nerve-sparing technique antegrade emission is preserved, and long term morbidity includes an abdominal scar and a 1% chance of latent small bowel obstruction. RPLND offers unique advantages over observation or adjuvant chemotherapy, including immediate pathologic staging, a simplified and less anxiety-prone follow-up involving less radiation exposure, and the potential for cure and the avoidance of chemotherapy for pathologic stage II patients.

1.6 Special considerations in stage I disease

1.6.1 Clinical stage I s patients

A small percentage of patients have elevated serum tumor markers which do not normalize appropriately following radical orchiectomy, despite an otherwise normal metastatic work-up, and are defined as clinical Stage I s disease. By virtue of the increased markers, these patients continue to harbor disease. While some have advocated RPLND in such situations, confinement of disease to the retroperitoneum is not assured, thus additional chemotherapy may be necessary should RPLND not affect cure. As a result, chemotherapy is recommended for Stage Is patients.

1.6.2 Chemoresistant pathology

A small subset of patients have adenocarcinoma, teratoma with malignant transformation (such as primitive neuroectodermal tumour (PNET)), or a sex chord stromal tumor in their orchiectomy specimen. These histologies are chemoresistant, and a subsequent relapse is unlikely to be responsive to chemotherapy. Thus, first line treatment should be RPLND.

1.7 Summary: Management options for clinical stage I non-seminomatous germ cell tumor of the testis

Appropriate treatment of Stage I NSGCT requires knowledge of the risk factors associated with recurrence, foresight regarding the likely outcomes and percentages associated with the three treatment strategies, the morbidities unique to each modality, and most importantly a keen understanding of a patient's desired approach to this complicated problem. Given that all three treatment modalities offer equivalent cure rates, a treatment strategy which focuses on minimizing overall morbidity, and approaches the problem in a manner which is synergistic with a patient's wishes, is most likely to be successful.

2. Management options for clinical stage II and III non-seminomatous germ cell tumor of the testis

Patients with clinical stage II disease have evidence of disease confined to their retroperitoneum following radical orchiectomy. Clinical stage III patients have disease outside of the retroperitoneum following orchiectomy. Patients with small volume (<5cm) stage II disease and normal serum tumor markers post-orchiectomy may be treated with either primary RPLND or induction chemotherapy. Patients with "bulky" stage II disease, those with persistently elevated serum tumor markers, and all patients with clinical stage III disease, require cisplatinum-based chemotherapy.

2.1 Primary RPLND for low volume clinical stage II disease

2.1.1 Clinical outcomes of primary RPLND

As with clinical stage I disease, primary RPLND in low volume clinical stage II disease is both a staging and a therapeutic procedure. Following RPLND, further treatment decisions are based upon the pathologic stage of disease, regardless of the initial *clinical* stage at presentation. Donohue reported on 174 clinical stage II patients undergoing full, bilateral primary RPLND from 1965 to 1989. (Donohue, Thornhill, Foster, Rowland, & Bihrle, 1995b) Interestingly, 23% of patients originally staged as CS II disease were shown to be pathologic stage I disease following primary RPLND. 65% of those patients who were pathologic stage II with a nodal mass of less than 5 cm were cured by RPLND alone – that is, did not receive adjuvant chemotherapy. Thus patients with clinical stage II disease who are proven to be pathologic stage II are cured at roughly the 70% level with surgery alone.

2.2 Induction chemotherapy for clinical stage II and III disease

2.2.1 Clinical outcomes of induction chemotherapy

All patients with persistently elevated tumor markers post orchiectomy and CS III patients should initially be treated with induction chemotherapy. Chemotherapy for germ cell tumors is cisplatinum-based, and the specific regimen is dictated by risk classification, using the International Germ Cell Cancer Consensus (IGCCC) classification system, which assigns risk based on the site of the primary tumor, post-orchiectomy serum tumor markers, and the site(s) of metastatic disease (Table 2). ("International Germ Cell Consensus Classification: a prognostic factor-based staging system for metastatic germ cell cancers. International Germ Cell Cancer Collaborative Group," 1997) Good risk patients are treated with 3 courses of bleomycin, etoposide, and cisplatinum (BEP). (Culine et al., 2007; Einhorn et al., 1989) In good risk patients over age 50 or with a strong smoking history, bleomycin may be omitted and 4 cycles of EP may be given instead. (Bosl et al., 1988; Culine, et al., 2007; Xiao et al., 1997) Standard therapy for intermediate and poor risk patients is 4 courses of BEP. Randomized trials evaluating high dose chemotherapy (HDCT) versus 4 cycles of BEP in poor risk patients as initial therapy failed to show an improved outcome in the HDCT arm. (Motzer et al., 2007) Overall, depending upon the patient population selected, roughly 70% of patients treated with induction chemotherapy for CS II or III disease will obtain a complete clinical response (CR) with normalization of serum tumor markers and complete radiographic resolution of all metastatic disease.

	Good Prognosis	Intermediate Prognosis	Poor Prognosis
Primary Site	Testis or Retroperitoneal	Testis or Retroperitoneal	Mediastinal
Metastases Site	No nonpulmonary visceral	No nonpulmonary visceral	Nonpulmonary visceral
Post Orchiectomy Serum Tumor Markers	AFP<1000 ng/mL βhCG<5000 IU/L LDH<1.5 x Normal upper limit	AFP 1-10,000 ng/mL βhcG 5-50,000IU/L LDH 1.5-10 x Normal upper limit	AFP>10,000 ng/mL βhCG>50,000 IU/L LDH>10 x Normal upper limit

Table 2. International Germ Cell Consensus Classification of Non Seminoma

2.3.1 Post-chemotherapy RPLND following complete response to induction chemotherapy

Following induction chemotherapy for CS II or III disease, patients achieving a CR are observed, as the risk of relapse is approximately 5%. (Ehrlich, Brames, Beck, Foster, & Einhorn, 2010) Recently, it has been shown that 20-25% of CR patients undergoing PC RPLND harbour microscopic teratoma in their retroperitoneum. (Karellas et al., 2007; Oldenburg et al., 2003) Thus there has emerged a controversy due to the disconnect between the pathologic finding of microscopic teratoma (20-25%) and clinically observed relapse rates (5%). The concern for physicians advocating immediate PC RPLND in this population is that with longer follow-up, the relapse rate will approach 20-25%. However, at 15 year follow-up, the relapse rate remains roughly 5%, thus the data continues to support surveillance as an appropriate strategy for CR patients.

2.3.2 PC RPLND for residual mass following induction chemotherapy

It is accepted worldwide that patients with normalization of serum tumor markers and persistent retroperitoneal mass following chemotherapy undergo PC RPLND. In this population, pathology reveals necrosis in 45%, teratoma in 45%, and active cancer in 10% (Toner et al., 1990).

For patients with necrosis at PC RPLND, surgery is a staging procedure only, and offers no therapeutic benefit. Relapse rates are approximately 5%, and no additional chemotherapy is required.

For patients with teratoma at PC RPLND, adjuvant chemotherapy is not given, as teratoma is chemotherapy insensitive. Nonetheless, teratoma at PC RPLND requires careful follow-up, as recurrence rates are not insignificant, and range from 5-20% with increasing size of mass. With a median post chemotherapy mass size of 3.0 cm, Memorial Sloan Kettering reported disease free survival of 83% at 5-years for resected teratoma. (Carver et al., 2007) In this study, patients with residual mass size less than 2 cm, 2 to 5 cm and > 5 cm had 5-year probabilities of freedom from recurrence of 94%, 91% and 59%, respectively ($p < 0.0005$). Other authors have had similar results. (Carver, et al., 2007; Loehrer et al., 1986; Svatek et al., 2009) Investigators from Indiana University recently reported recurrence rates after resection of large volume (> 10 cm) teratoma. (S. D.W. Beck, Foster, Bihrle, Donohue, & Einhorn, 2007) The 2 and 5-year recurrence free survival for the 99 patients was 86% and 75%, with a mean follow up of 42 months, suggesting that in large volume masses, recurrence rates are also noteworthy. As a result, follow-up of teratoma at PC RPLND need include serial abdominal CT scan.

The presence of active cancer at PC RPLND portends a poor prognosis, and it has been standard practice to give two courses of adjuvant chemotherapy. In this population, Spiess reported the 5 year disease-free survival rate to be 50%. (Spiess et al., 2007) An international study group on testis cancer reported the outcomes of 238 patients with active cancer at PC RPLND. Variables predictive of survival included incomplete surgery, viable malignant cells > 10% of surgical specimen, and poor or intermediate IGCCC risk category. (Fizazi et al., 2001)Patients with no adverse factors experienced a 5-year progression free survival of 90% compared to 41% for 2 or more risk factors. Furthermore, on multivariate analysis postoperative chemotherapy was associated with a significantly better progression free survival ($p < 0.001$), but not overall survival ($p = 0.26$). Thus, while adjuvant chemotherapy does not improve overall survival, it does reduce recurrence rates to 30%, and thereby avoids the morbidity of second line chemotherapy for those who do not recur.

2.3.3 Follow-up after PC RPLND

PC RPLND follow-up is based upon retroperitoneal pathology. Patients with necrosis are at low risk of relapse, and follow-up should include physical exam, serial chest imaging and serum tumor markers. Routine abdominal imaging is not necessary in this population. In addition to the routine follow-up necessary for necrosis, patients with teratoma are at some risk of retroperitoneal relapse, and therefore require serial abdominal CT scans. Follow-up for active cancer should be tailored individually, though will include physical exam, serum tumor markers, chest X-ray and abdominal imaging.

2.3.4 Summary: Induction chemotherapy and PC RPLND

Following induction chemotherapy for clinical stage II or III disease, patients with a complete response to chemotherapy are most commonly managed with observation. Patients with a persistent retroperitoneal mass and negative serum tumor markers routinely undergo PC RPLND. 45% of PC RPLND patients will harbor necrosis, with a relapse rate of 5%. 45% harbor teratoma with relapses ranging from 5-20%, depending on mass size. The 10% of patients with active cancer in their retroperitoneum at PC RPLND are treated with adjuvant chemotherapy to improve disease-free survival. Adjuvant chemotherapy has yet to demonstrate improved overall survival in this population.

2.4 Special considerations in stage II and III disease

2.4.1 Induction chemotherapy failure

Patients with disease relapse or disease progression despite first line chemotherapy are candidates for salvage therapy. Disease progression may be identified by persistently elevated tumor markers or increasing mass size. A minority of such patients will have anatomically confined disease that is amenable to surgical resection, and may undergo "desperation surgery". (S. D. Beck, Foster, Bihrle, Einhorn, & Donohue, 2005; Murphy et al., 1993) For the remaining patients with multifocal disease, treatment options include salvage chemotherapy with cisplatin plus ifosfamide plus vinblastine, (Loehrer, Gonin, Nichols, Weathers, & Einhorn, 1998) or paclitaxel (Motzer, Sheinfeld, et al., 2000) for four courses, or high-dose chemotherapy with autologous hematopoietic stem-cell transplantation to rescue the bone marrow from the myeloablative effect of chemotherapy. (Einhorn et al., 2007; Motzer, Mazumdar, et al., 2000; Rick et al., 1998)

2.4.2 Determining the extent of dissection at PC RPLND

Many patients from the 1970's and 1980's undergoing post chemotherapy surgery had high volume residual disease and the decision to perform a full, bilateral RPLND was therefore rational and appropriate. Since chemotherapy is now being administered for relatively low volume retroperitoneal disease, and since these tumors are typically restricted to the primary landing zone of the affected testicle, the question has arisen as to the appropriateness of full bilateral PC RPLND in this population.

Proponents of modified dissections note that with appropriate patient selection, the risk of extra-template disease and its clinical significance is low. In 1992, investigators from Memorial Sloan-Kettering published a series of 113 patients undergoing full bilateral PC RPLND, with an 8% incidence of disease (cancer/teratoma) identified in the contralateral landing zone. (D. P. Wood, Jr., Herr, Heller, et al., 1992) This cohort all presented with "bulky disease", and were treated with cisplatin- or carboplatin-based chemotherapy. Based upon these findings, the authors concluded that a modified dissection should be considered in patients with 1) no palpable residual tumor mass, 2) a left primary tumor, or 3) a right primary tumor and no evidence of cancer/teratoma on frozen section analysis of the residual mass. Fossa et al. reported the results of 87 patients with residual masses less than 20 mm undergoing modified PC RPLND. (Oldenburg, et al., 2003) Pathology revealed necrosis in 67%, teratoma in 26%, and cancer in 7%. Five relapses occurred in this study, with no recurrences in the retroperitoneum, indicating that the template of dissection was adequate. Indiana University recently reported outcomes of 100 patients undergoing a modified post chemotherapy dissection. (S.D.W. Beck, Foster, Bihrle, & Donohue, 2005) The selection criteria included low-volume retroperitoneal disease (< 5 cm) both pre- and postchemotherapy, restricted to the primary landing zone of the affected testicle. Pathology revealed cancer in 2%, teratoma in 62% and necrosis in 36%. Three patients relapsed, all outside the boundaries of a full bilateral dissection, and the 2-year progression free survival was 95%. Others have also demonstrated the safety of a modified PC RPLND in select patients, (Ehrlich, Yossepowitch, Kedar, & Baniel, 2006; Rabbani et al., 1998) thus it appears that a modified dissection may be appropriate in select patients.

Though limited dissection is appropriate in a subset of patients, the vast majority of patients undergoing PC RPLND require a full, bilateral dissection.

2.4.3 Complicated PC RPLND

Complicated PC RPLND is defined as: 1) PC RPLND after more than induction chemotherapy ("salvage RPLND"), PC RPLND after previous RPLND ("redo RPLND"), or PC RPLND in the setting of persistently elevated markers or progression of disease after chemotherapy ("desperation RPLND"). (Donohue, et al., 1998)

Indiana University reported the outcomes of patients undergoing "complicated" RPLND. The incidence of active cancer at "salvage" RPLND was 50%, with an overall survival of 50% to 60%. There appeared to be no benefit with adjuvant chemotherapy in this population. Overall survival for the 188 patients undergoing "redo" surgery was 63%. Memorial Sloan-Kettering reported a 67% 5-year disease specific survival for 57 patients undergoing redo surgery. (McKiernan et al., 2003) Historically, persistent serum tumor marker elevation after chemotherapy has been considered a relative contraindication to surgery, due to supposed systemic disease and low chance of cure with local therapy alone. These "desperation" patients were therefore treated with salvage chemotherapy. Over the last 15 years, however, several centers have experienced surgical cures in this population. (S. D. Beck, R. S. Foster, R. Bihrle, L. H. Einhorn, et al., 2005; Eastham, Wilson, Russell, Ahlering, & Skinner, 1994; Murphy, et al., 1993; D. P. Wood, Jr., Herr, Motzer, et al., 1992) Thus, a subset of patients with elevated serum tumor markers after chemotherapy are curable with surgery. Approximately 50% of patients undergoing post chemotherapy surgery with elevated serum tumor markers are alive at 5-years. Half of these patients are found to harbor viable non-teratomatous germ cell tumor, and a third of these are alive at 5-years. Interestingly, this small subset population observes no benefit from adjuvant chemotherapy. Clearly, there is a role for surgery in selected patients with elevated serum tumor markers. The decision to proceed with surgery *in lieu* of second or third line chemotherapy involves identifying patients that are unlikely to obtain a complete response with systemic therapy, are of acceptable surgical candidacy, are harboring resectable tumors which could potentially be curable with negative margins, and following resection are offered acceptable morbidity profiles.

2.4.4 Surgical management of pulmonary extraperitoneal disease

Selection of patients for pulmonary resection typically includes patients with residual lung nodules and normal serum tumor markers after chemotherapy. Much like PC RPLND, resection of residual teratoma or active cancer in the pulmonary system can be therapeutic and therefore the morbidity of thoracotomy is justified. Conversely, resection of residual necrosis is a staging procedure only.

Efforts to predict pulmonary histology prior to surgical resection have been somewhat successful. Excluding series with less than 100 patients, there are 2 retrospective studies identifying variables predictive of pulmonary histology. Tognini et al reviewed 143 post chemotherapy patients who underwent resection of residual retroperitoneal and chest disease under the same anesthetic. (Tognoni et al., 1998) Pathologic concordance between pulmonary and retroperitoneal masses existed in 77.5% of patients with necrosis, 70% with teratoma, and 69% with active cancer. For surgery-naïve patients experiencing normalization of tumor markers following first line chemotherapy, a pathologic concordance between pulmonary and retroperitoneal masses of 86% for patients with necrosis was seen. An international, multicenter, retrospective review evaluated the concordance of retroperitoneal and pulmonary histology in 215 patients. (Steyerberg et al., 1997) The strongest predictor of pulmonary histology was the histology found at PC RPLND -- if PC RPLND histology revealed necrosis, the probability of necrosis at thoracotomy was 89%.

As such, patients with small pulmonary nodules may be observed with serial chest imaging. Masses which enlarge on observation are thus identified, and represent the small proportion of patients with residual disease in the form of teratoma (5%) or active cancer (1-4%). Such patients could conceivably then undergo surgical resection without a decrease in their expected survival rate. In fact, in subgroups with pulmonary nodules and necrosis in the retroperitoneum, such an approach would spare more than 90% of patients the morbidity of thoracotomy.

There is no data comparing immediate resection of residual pulmonary nodules versus delayed resection upon progression. Decision-making with regard to residual pulmonary mass resection must take into account technical feasibility, patient morbidity and potential benefit, future access to health care, and of course patient preference.

2.4.5 Surgical management of nonpulmonary extraperitoneal disease

NSGCT metastatic to extraperitoneal sites beyond the pulmonary system are quite rare, and require specific site-based therapeutic approaches.

Residual post-chemotherapy mediastinal or neck masses are typically removed either at time of RPLND or as a staged procedure.

Brain metastases occur in 1% of patients, and Cisplatin-based chemotherapy is recommended as initial therapy in patients with brain metastases at initial presentation. Balmaceda et al reported a 57% complete response rate in 68 patients with brain involvement with chemotherapy alone. (Balmaceda et al., 1996) Surgical resection should be considered for residual disease. Radiotherapy does not appear to influence survival in this select population, and confers considerable morbidity by way of declining functional cognitive status.

Indiana University demonstrated that approximately 70% of resected liver lesions are necrosis and the histologic concordance between retroperitoneal histology and liver histology is 94.4% for necrosis, 25.9% for teratoma and 38.5% for active cancer. (Jacobsen et al.) With this data in mind, observation of liver metastases should be considered when retroperitoneal histology reveals necrosis or when the volume and/or location of the hepatic involvement require a significant surgical undertaking. If the mass enlarges on surveillance, then surgery or second-line chemotherapy should be considered.

2.4.6 Management of late relapse

Late relapse of testis cancer is defined as recurrence of disease later than 2 years after initial successful treatment. In a pooled analysis of 5880 patients, late relapse occurred in 119 of 3704 (3.2%) patients with non-seminoma. The retroperitoneum is the predominant site of relapse, followed by the lung, and 70% present with an elevated AFP. About 40% to 50% of patients with late relapse are curable, predominantly through surgery, as these tumors are by and large chemoresistant. (Baniel, et al., 1995; George et al., 2003)

2.5 Summary: Management options for clinical stage II and III non-seminomatous germ cell tumor of the testis

Patients with low-volume clinical stage II disease with normal serum tumor markers may undergo primary RPLND *in lieu* of systemic chemotherapy. Surgery alone without chemotherapy can cure 50-70% of patients with pathologic stage II disease. The remainder are cured with chemotherapy at relapse.

Patients with elevated serum tumor markers, bulky clinical stage II disease, and all clinical stage III patients require induction chemotherapy. 70% of these patients will achieve CR, and these patients are observed, as the relapse rate is less than 5%. Patients with normalization of serum tumor markers and a persistent retroperitoneal mass routinely require PC RPLND. Outcome is dependent upon pathology.

Patients with more complicated disease require individualized therapy, which may involve salvage chemotherapy, surgery, or both. Relapses occurring more than two years since last treatment are best approached with surgery. Patients requiring "complicated" PC RPLND, presenting with late relapse, or harboring extraperitoneal disease are candidates for referral to tertiary centers of considerable experience in these difficult scenarios.

3. Explanation of terms and abbreviations

Adjuvant Chemotherapy - A term denoting chemotherapy that is administered after first receiving definitive local therapy (such as surgery). This second therapy is given to patients under the assumption that micrometastatic disease persists despite the initial local therapy.

CT A & P - Computed Tomography Scan of the Abdomen and Pelvis. Providing detailed information about the size and location of potential sites of metastatic testis cancer in the abdomen and pelvis, these scans are the pelvic imaging modality of choice for surveillance and investigation of nonseminomatous germs cell tumors.

CXR - Chest X-ray. A chest imaging modality for the surveillance and investigation of patients with nonseminomatous germ cell tumors of the testis.

Induction Chemotherapy - A term denoting chemotherapy that is administered as initial treatment where disease is too advanced for other modalities (such as surgery).

IVC - Inferior Vena Cava. Anatomical term for large vein coursing through retroperitoneum, returning venous blood to the right atrium. Metastatic testis cancer frequently intimately involved with this structure.

PC RPLND - Post-chemotherapy retroperitoneal lymph node dissection. Surgical procedure to remove all lymphatic tissue in the retroperitoneal space which lies between the ureters, superior to the common iliac vessels, and inferior to the crus of the diaphragm, performed after patient has received chemotherapy.

RPLND - Retroperitoneal lymph node dissection. Surgical procedure to remove all lymphatic tissue in the retroperitoneal space which lies between the ureters, superior to the common iliac vessels, and inferior to the crus of the diaphragm.

Salvage Chemotherapy - A term denoting chemotherapy given after relapse or progression of disease, despite prior induction chemotherapy

STM - Serum tumor markers. In nonseminomatous germ cell tumor of the testis, the most important markers are alpha fetoprotein (AFP), the beta subunit of human chorionic gonadotropin (βhCG) and lactate dehydrogenase (LDH). These proteins are easily isolated from blood samples, and are highly reliable in terms of their ability to quantify disease burden and/or assess response to therapy.

4. References

Abdel-Aziz, K. F., Anderson, J. K., Svatek, R., Margulis, V., Sagalowsky, A. I., & Cadeddu, J. A. (2006). Laparoscopic and open retroperitoneal lymph-node dissection for clinical stage I nonseminomatous germ-cell testis tumors. *J Endourol, 20*(9), 627-631.

Albers, P., Siener, R., Krege, S., Schmelz, H. U., Dieckmann, K. P., Heidenreich, A., . . . Hartmann, M. (2008). Randomized phase III trial comparing retroperitoneal lymph node dissection with one course of bleomycin and etoposide plus cisplatin chemotherapy in the adjuvant treatment of clinical stage I Nonseminomatous testicular germ cell tumors: AUO trial AH 01/94 by the German Testicular Cancer Study Group. *J Clin Oncol, 26*(18), 2966-2972.

Albqami, N., & Janetschek, G. (2005). Laparoscopic retroperitoneal lymph-node dissection in the management of clinical stage I and II testicular cancer. *J Endourol, 19*(6), 683-692; discussion 692.

Balmaceda, C., Heller, G., Rosenblum, M., Diez, B., Villablanca, J. G., Kellie, S., . . . Finlay, J. L. (1996). Chemotherapy without irradiation--a novel approach for newly diagnosed CNS germ cell tumors: results of an international cooperative trial. The First International Central Nervous System Germ Cell Tumor Study. *J Clin Oncol, 14*(11), 2908-2915.

Baniel, J., Foster, R. S., Gonin, R., Messemer, J. E., Donohue, J. P., & Einhorn, L. H. (1995). Late relapse of testicular cancer. *J Clin Oncol, 13*(5), 1170-1176.

Baniel, J., Foster, R. S., Rowland, R. G., Bihrle, R., & Donohue, J. P. (1994). Complications of primary retroperitoneal lymph node dissection. *J Urol, 152*(2 Pt 1), 424-427.

Beck, S. D., Bey, A. L., Bihrle, R., & Foster, R. S. (2010). Ejaculatory status and fertility rates after primary retroperitoneal lymph node dissection. *J Urol, 184*(5), 2078-2080.

Beck, S. D., Foster, R. S., Bihrle, R., Cheng, L., & Donohue, J. P. (2005). Does the histology of nodal metastasis predict systemic relapse after retroperitoneal lymph node dissection in pathological stage B1 germ cell tumors? *J Urol, 174*(4 Pt 1), 1287-1290; discussion 1290.

Beck, S. D., Foster, R. S., Bihrle, R., Cheng, L., Ulbright, T. M., & Donohue, J. P. (2005). Impact of the number of positive lymph nodes on disease-free survival in patients with pathological stage B1 nonseminomatous germ cell tumor. *J Urol, 174*(1), 143-145.

Beck, S. D., Foster, R. S., Bihrle, R., Einhorn, L. H., & Donohue, J. P. (2005). Outcome analysis for patients with elevated serum tumor markers at postchemotherapy retroperitoneal lymph node dissection. *J Clin Oncol, 23*(25), 6149-6156.

Beck, S. D.W., Foster, R.S., Bihrle, R., Donohue, J.P., & Einhorn, L. H. (2007). Long term outcomes for patients with high volume retroperitoneal teratoma undergoing post chemotherpay surgery. *Journal of Urology, Abstract, 177*, 331.

Beck, S.D.W., Foster, R. S., Bihrle, R., & Donohue, J. P. (2005). Is full bilateral retroperitoneal lymph node dissection always necessary for post chemotherapy resdual tumor? *AUA, San Antonia Texas, Abstract.*

Beck, S.D.W., Peterson, M.D., Foster, R. S., Bihrle, R., & Donohue, J. P. (2006). What is the short-term morbidity of primary retroperitoneal lymph node dissection in a contemporary group of patients? *American Urologic Association*(Abstract), .

Behnia, M., Foster, R., Einhorn, L. H., Donohue, J., & Nichols, C. R. (2000). Adjuvant bleomycin, etoposide and cisplatin in pathological stage II non-seminomatous testicular cancer. the Indiana University experience. *Eur J Cancer, 36*(4), 472-475.

Bosl, G. J., Geller, N. L., Bajorin, D., Leitner, S. P., Yagoda, A., Golbey, R. B., . . . et al. (1988). A randomized trial of etoposide + cisplatin versus vinblastine + bleomycin + cisplatin + cyclophosphamide + dactinomycin in patients with good-prognosis germ cell tumors. *J Clin Oncol, 6*(8), 1231-1238.

Brenner, D. J., & Hall, E. J. (2007). Computed tomography--an increasing source of radiation exposure. *N Engl J Med, 357*(22), 2277-2284. doi: 357/22/2277 [pii] 10.1056/NEJMra072149

Brydoy, M., Oldenburg, J., Klepp, O., Bremnes, R. M., Wist, E. A., Wentzel-Larsen, T., . . . Fossa, S. D. (2009). Observational study of prevalence of long-term Raynaud-like phenomena and neurological side effects in testicular cancer survivors. *J Natl Cancer Inst, 101*(24), 1682-1695.

Carver, B. S., Shayegan, B., Serio, A., Motzer, R. J., Bosl, G. J., & Sheinfeld, J. (2007). Long-term clinical outcome after postchemotherapy retroperitoneal lymph node dissection in men with residual teratoma. *J Clin Oncol, 25*(9), 1033-1037.

Chevreau, C., Mazerolles, C., Soulie, M., Gaspard, M. H., Mourey, L., Bujan, L., . . . Malavaud, B. (2004). Long-term efficacy of two cycles of BEP regimen in high-risk stage I nonseminomatous testicular germ cell tumors with embryonal carcinoma and/or vascular invasion. *Eur Urol, 46*(2), 209-214; discussion 214-205.

Colls, B. M., Harvey, V. J., Skelton, L., Frampton, C. M., Thompson, P. I., Bennett, M., . . . Kennedy, I. C. (1999). Late results of surveillance of clinical stage I nonseminoma germ cell testicular tumours: 17 years' experience in a national study in New Zealand. *BJU Int, 83*(1), 76-82.

Culine, S., Kerbrat, P., Kramar, A., Theodore, C., Chevreau, C., Geoffrois, L., . . . Droz, J. P. (2007). Refining the optimal chemotherapy regimen for good-risk metastatic nonseminomatous germ-cell tumors: a randomized trial of the Genito-Urinary Group of the French Federation of Cancer Centers (GETUG T93BP). *Ann Oncol, 18*(5), 917-924. doi: mdm062 [pii] 10.1093/annonc/mdm062

Culine, S., Theodore, C., Farhat, F., Bekradda, M., Terrier-Lacombe, M. J., & Droz, J. P. (1996). Cisplatin-based chemotherapy after retroperitoneal lymph node dissection in patients with pathological stage II nonseminomatous germ cell tumors. *J Surg Oncol, 61*(3), 195-198.

Cullen, M. H., Stenning, S. P., Parkinson, M. C., Fossa, S. D., Kaye, S. B., Horwich, A. H., . . . Jakes, R. (1996). Short-course adjuvant chemotherapy in high-risk stage I nonseminomatous germ cell tumors of the testis: a Medical Research Council report. *J Clin Oncol, 14*(4), 1106-1113.

Divrik, R. T., Akdogan, B., Ozen, H., & Zorlu, F. (2006). Outcomes of surveillance protocol of clinical stage I nonseminomatous germ cell tumors-is shift to risk adapted policy justified? *J Urol, 176*(4 Pt 1), 1424-1429; discussion 1429-1430.

Donohue, J. P., Thornhill, J. A., Foster, R. S., Rowland, R. G., & Bihrle, R. (1993a). Primary retroperitoneal lymph node dissection in clinical stage A non-seminomatous germ cell testis cancer. Review of the Indiana University experience 1965-1989. *Br J Urol, 71*(3), 326-335.

Donohue, J. P., Thornhill, J. A., Foster, R. S., Rowland, R. G., & Bihrle, R. (1993b). Retroperitoneal lymphadenectomy for clinical stage A testis cancer (1965 to 1989): modifications of technique and impact on ejaculation. *J Urol, 149*(2), 237-243.

Donohue, J. P., Thornhill, J. A., Foster, R. S., Rowland, R. G., & Bihrle, R. (1993c). Retroperitoneal lymphadenectomy for clinical stage A testis cancer (1965 to 1989): modifications of technique and impact on ejaculation. *J Urol, 149*(2), 237-243.

Donohue, J. P., Thornhill, J. A., Foster, R. S., Rowland, R. G., & Bihrle, R. (1995a). Clinical stage B non-seminomatous germ cell testis cancer: the Indiana University experience (1965-1989) using routine primary retroperitoneal lymph node dissection. *Eur J Cancer, 31A*(10), 1599-1604.

Donohue, J. P., Thornhill, J. A., Foster, R. S., Rowland, R. G., & Bihrle, R. (1995b). Clinical stage B non-seminomatous germ cell testis cancer: the Indiana University experience (1965-1989) using routine primary retroperitoneal lymph node dissection. *Eur J Cancer, 31A*(10), 1599-1604.

Eastham, J. A., Wilson, T. G., Russell, C., Ahlering, T. E., & Skinner, D. G. (1994). Surgical resection in patients with nonseminomatous germ cell tumor who fail to normalize serum tumor markers after chemotherapy. *Urology, 43*(1), 74-80.

Ehrlich, Y., Brames, M. J., Beck, S. D., Foster, R. S., & Einhorn, L. H. (2010). Long-term follow-up of Cisplatin combination chemotherapy in patients with disseminated nonseminomatous germ cell tumors: is a postchemotherapy retroperitoneal lymph node dissection needed after complete remission? *J Clin Oncol, 28*(4), 531-536. doi: JCO.2009.23.0714 [pii] 10.1200/JCO.2009.23.0714

Ehrlich, Y., Yossepowitch, O., Kedar, D., & Baniel, J. (2006). Distribution of nodal metastases after chemotherapy in nonseminomatous testis cancer: a possible indication for limited dissection. *BJU Int, 97*(6), 1221-1224.

Einhorn, L. H., Williams, S. D., Chamness, A., Brames, M. J., Perkins, S. M., & Abonour, R. (2007). High-dose chemotherapy and stem-cell rescue for metastatic germ-cell tumors. *N Engl J Med, 357*(4), 340-348.

Einhorn, L. H., Williams, S. D., Loehrer, P. J., Birch, R., Drasga, R., Omura, G., & Greco, F. A. (1989). Evaluation of optimal duration of chemotherapy in favorable-prognosis disseminated germ cell tumors: a Southeastern Cancer Study Group protocol. *J Clin Oncol, 7*(3), 387-391.

Fizazi, K., Tjulandin, S., Salvioni, R., Germa-Lluch, J. R., Bouzy, J., Ragan, D., . . . Mahe, C. (2001). Viable malignant cells after primary chemotherapy for disseminated nonseminomatous germ cell tumors: prognostic factors and role of postsurgery chemotherapy--results from an international study group. *J Clin Oncol, 19*(10), 2647-2657.

Foster, R. S., McNulty, A., Rubin, L. R., Bennett, R., Rowland, R. G., Sledge, G. W., . . . Donohue, J. P. (1994). Fertility considerations in nerve-sparing retroperitoneal lymph-node dissection. *World J Urol, 12*(3), 136-138.

Freedman, L. S., Parkinson, M. C., Jones, W. G., Oliver, R. T., Peckham, M. J., Read, G., . . . Williams, C. J. (1987). Histopathology in the prediction of relapse of patients with stage I testicular teratoma treated by orchidectomy alone. *Lancet, 2*(8554), 294-298.

Gels, M. E., Hoekstra, H. J., Sleijfer, D. T., Marrink, J., de Bruijn, H. W., Molenaar, W. M., . . . Schraffordt Koops, H. (1995). Detection of recurrence in patients with clinical stage I nonseminomatous testicular germ cell tumors and consequences for further follow-up: a single-center 10-year experience. *J Clin Oncol, 13*(5), 1188-1194.

George, D. W., Foster, R. S., Hromas, R. A., Robertson, K. A., Vance, G. H., Ulbright, T. M., . . . Einhorn, L. H. (2003). Update on late relapse of germ cell tumor: a clinical and molecular analysis. *J Clin Oncol, 21*(1), 113-122.

Gerl, A., Clemm, C., Kohl, P., & al., et. (1994). Adjuvant chemotherapy of stage II non-seminomatous germ cell tumors. *Oncol Rep*(1), 209-212.

Groll, R. J., Warde, P., & Jewett, M. A. (2007). A comprehensive systematic review of testicular germ cell tumor surveillance. *Crit Rev Oncol Hematol, 64*(3), 182-197. doi: S1040-8428(07)00109-6 [pii] 10.1016/j.critrevonc.2007.04.014

Hao, D., Seidel, J., Brant, R., Alexander, F., Ernst, D. S., Summers, N., . . . Stewart, D. A. (1998). Compliance of clinical stage I nonseminomatous germ cell tumor patients with surveillance. *J Urol, 160*(3 Pt 1), 768-771.

Heidenreich, A., Albers, P., Hartmann, M., Kliesch, S., Kohrmann, K. U., Krege, S., . . . Weissbach, L. (2003). Complications of primary nerve sparing retroperitoneal lymph node dissection for clinical stage I nonseminomatous germ cell tumors of the testis: experience of the German Testicular Cancer Study Group. *J Urol, 169*(5), 1710-1714.

Herr, H. W., Bar-Chama, N., O'Sullivan, M., & Sogani, P. C. (1998). Paternity in men with stage I testis tumors on surveillance. *J Clin Oncol, 16*(2), 733-734.

Huddart, R. A., Norman, A., Shahidi, M., Horwich, A., Coward, D., Nicholls, J., & Dearnaley, D. P. (2003). Cardiovascular disease as a long-term complication of treatment for testicular cancer. *J Clin Oncol, 21*(8), 1513-1523.

Huyghe, E., Matsuda, T., Daudin, M., Chevreau, C., Bachaud, J. M., Plante, P., . . . Thonneau, P. (2004). Fertility after testicular cancer treatments: results of a large multicenter study. *Cancer, 100*(4), 732-737. doi: 10.1002/cncr.11950

International Germ Cell Consensus Classification: a prognostic factor-based staging system for metastatic germ cell cancers. International Germ Cell Cancer Collaborative Group. (1997). *J Clin Oncol, 15*(2), 594-603.

Jacobsen, N. E., Beck, S. D., Jacobson, L. E., Bihrle, R., Einhorn, L. H., & Foster, R. S. Is retroperitoneal histology predictive of liver histology at concurrent post-chemotherapy retroperitoneal lymph node dissection and hepatic resection? *J Urol, 184*(3), 949-953.

Janetschek, G., Hobisch, A., Holtl, L., & Bartsch, G. (1996). Retroperitoneal lymphadenectomy for clinical stage I nonseminomatous testicular tumor: laparoscopy versus open surgery and impact of learning curve. *J Urol, 156*(1), 89-93; discussion 94.

Jewett, M. A. (1990). Nerve-sparing technique for retroperitoneal lymphadenectomy in testis cancer. *Urol Clin North Am, 17*(2), 449-456.

Kakehi, Y., Kamoto, T., Kawakita, M., & Ogawa, O. (2002). Follow-up of clinical stage I testicular cancer patients: cost and risk benefit considerations. *Int J Urol, 9*(3), 154-160; discussion 160-151.

Kakiashvili, D. M., Zuniga, A., & Jewett, M. A. (2009). High risk NSGCT: case for surveillance. *World J Urol, 27*(4), 441-447.

Karellas, M, Carver, B. S., Stasi, J., Motzer, R. J., Bosl, G. J., & Sheinfeld, J. (2007). Clinical outcome following post-chemotherapy retroperitoneal lymph node dissection for the with CII non-seminomatous germ cell tumors and a radiographically normal retroperitoneum. [Abstract]. *J Urol, 177*(4), 277.

Kennedy, B. J., Torkelson, J. L., & Fraley, E. E. (1994). Adjuvant chemotherapy for stage II nonseminomatous germ cell cancer of the testis. *Cancer, 73*(5), 1485-1489.

Kenney, P. A., & Tuerk, I. A. (2008). Complications of laparoscopic retroperitoneal lymph node dissection in testicular cancer. *World J Urol, 26*(6), 561-569.

Kollmannsberger, C., Moore, C., Chi, K. N., Murray, N., Daneshmand, S., Gleave, M., . . . Nichols, C. R. (2010). Non-risk-adapted surveillance for patients with stage I nonseminomatous testicular germ-cell tumors: diminishing treatment-related morbidity while maintaining efficacy. *Ann Oncol, 21*(6), 1296-1301. doi: mdp473 [pii] 10.1093/annonc/mdp473

Kondagunta, G. V., Sheinfeld, J., Mazumdar, M., Mariani, T. V., Bajorin, D., Bacik, J., . . . Motzer, R. J. (2004). Relapse-free and overall survival in patients with pathologic stage II nonseminomatous germ cell cancer treated with etoposide and cisplatin adjuvant chemotherapy. *J Clin Oncol, 22*(3), 464-467.

Loehrer, P. J., Sr., Gonin, R., Nichols, C. R., Weathers, T., & Einhorn, L. H. (1998). Vinblastine plus ifosfamide plus cisplatin as initial salvage therapy in recurrent germ cell tumor. *J Clin Oncol, 16*(7), 2500-2504.

Loehrer, P. J., Sr., Hui, S., Clark, S., Seal, M., Einhorn, L. H., Williams, S. D., . . . Donohue, J. P. (1986). Teratoma following cisplatin-based combination chemotherapy for nonseminomatous germ cell tumors: a clinicopathological correlation. *J Urol, 135*(6), 1183-1189.

Maroto, P., Garcia del Muro, X., Aparicio, J., Paz-Ares, L., Arranz, J. A., Guma, J., . . . Germa-Lluch, J. R. (2005). Multicentre risk-adapted management for stage I non-seminomatous germ cell tumours. *Ann Oncol, 16*(12), 1915-1920.

McKiernan, J. M., Motzer, R. J., Bajorin, D. F., Bacik, J., Bosl, G. J., & Sheinfeld, J. (2003). Reoperative retroperitoneal surgery for nonseminomatous germ cell tumor: clinical presentation, patterns of recurrence, and outcome. *Urology, 62*(4), 732-736.

Meinke, A. H., 3rd, Estes, N. C., & Ernst, C. B. (1979). Chylous ascites following abdominal aortic aneurysmectomy. Management with total parenteral hyperalimentation. *Ann Surg, 190*(5), 631-633.

Motzer, R. J., Mazumdar, M., Sheinfeld, J., Bajorin, D. F., Macapinlac, H. A., Bains, M., . . . Bosl, G. J. (2000). Sequential dose-intensive paclitaxel, ifosfamide, carboplatin, and etoposide salvage therapy for germ cell tumor patients. *J Clin Oncol, 18*(6), 1173-1180.

Motzer, R. J., Nichols, C. J., Margolin, K. A., Bacik, J., Richardson, P. G., Vogelzang, N. J., . . . Bosl, G. J. (2007). Phase III randomized trial of conventional-dose chemotherapy with or without high-dose chemotherapy and autologous hematopoietic stem-cell rescue as first-line treatment for patients with poor-prognosis metastatic germ cell tumors. *J Clin Oncol, 25*(3), 247-256. doi: 25/3/247 [pii] 10.1200/JCO.2005.05.4528

Motzer, R. J., Sheinfeld, J., Mazumdar, M., Bains, M., Mariani, T., Bacik, J., . . . Bosl, G. J. (2000). Paclitaxel, ifosfamide, and cisplatin second-line therapy for patients with relapsed testicular germ cell cancer. *J Clin Oncol, 18*(12), 2413-2418.

Murphy, B. R., Breeden, E. S., Donohue, J. P., Messemer, J., Walsh, W., Roth, B. J., & Einhorn, L. H. (1993). Surgical salvage of chemorefractory germ cell tumors. *J Clin Oncol, 11*(2), 324-329.

Oldenburg, J., Alfsen, G. C., Lien, H. H., Aass, N., Waehre, H., & Fossa, S. D. (2003). Postchemotherapy retroperitoneal surgery remains necessary in patients with nonseminomatous testicular cancer and minimal residual tumor masses. *J Clin Oncol, 21*(17), 3310-3317.

Oliver, R. T., Raja, M. A., Ong, J., & Gallagher, C. J. (1992). Pilot study to evaluate impact of a policy of adjuvant chemotherapy for high risk stage 1 malignant teratoma on overall relapse rate of stage 1 cancer patients. *J Urol, 148*(5), 1453-1455; discussion 1455-1456.

Rabbani, F., Goldenberg, S. L., Gleave, M. E., Paterson, R. F., Murray, N., & Sullivan, L. D. (1998). Retroperitoneal lymphadenectomy for post-chemotherapy residual masses: is a modified dissection and resection of residual masses sufficient? *Br J Urol, 81*(2), 295-300.

Rabbani, F., Sheinfeld, J., Farivar-Mohseni, H., Leon, A., Rentzepis, M. J., Reuter, V. E., . . . Bosl, G. J. (2001). Low-volume nodal metastases detected at retroperitoneal lymphadenectomy for testicular cancer: pattern and prognostic factors for relapse. *J Clin Oncol, 19*(7), 2020-2025.

Raghavan, D., Colls, B., Levi, J., Fitzharris, B., Tattersall, M. H., Atkinson, C., . . . Wines, R. (1988). Surveillance for stage I non-seminomatous germ cell tumours of the testis: the optimal protocol has not yet been defined. *Br J Urol, 61*(6), 522-526.

Rassweiler, J. J., Scheitlin, W., Heidenreich, A., Laguna, M. P., & Janetschek, G. (2008). Laparoscopic retroperitoneal lymph node dissection: does it still have a role in the management of clinical stage I nonseminomatous testis cancer? A European perspective. *Eur Urol, 54*(5), 1004-1015.

Read, G., Stenning, S. P., Cullen, M. H., Parkinson, M. C., Horwich, A., Kaye, S. B., & Cook, P. A. (1992). Medical Research Council prospective study of surveillance for stage I testicular teratoma. Medical Research Council Testicular Tumors Working Party. *J Clin Oncol, 10*(11), 1762-1768.

Richie, J. P., & Kantoff, P. W. (1991). Is adjuvant chemotherapy necessary for patients with stage B1 testicular cancer? *J Clin Oncol, 9*(8), 1393-1396.

Rick, O., Beyer, J., Kingreen, D., Schwella, N., Krusch, A., Schleicher, J., . . . Siegert, W. (1998). High-dose chemotherapy in germ cell tumours: a large single centre experience. *Eur J Cancer, 34*(12), 1883-1888.

Rustin, G. J., Mead, G. M., Stenning, S. P., Vasey, P. A., Aass, N., Huddart, R. A., . . . Kirk, S. J. (2007). Randomized trial of two or five computed tomography scans in the surveillance of patients with stage I nonseminomatous germ cell tumors of the testis: Medical Research Council Trial TE08, ISRCTN56475197--the National Cancer Research Institute Testis Cancer Clinical Studies Group. *J Clin Oncol, 25*(11), 1310-1315.

Sagstuen, H., Aass, N., Fossa, S. D., Dahl, O., Klepp, O., Wist, E. A., . . . Bremnes, R. M. (2005). Blood pressure and body mass index in long-term survivors of testicular cancer. *J Clin Oncol, 23*(22), 4980-4990.

Spiess, P. E., Tannir, N. M., Tu, S. M., Brown, G. A., Liu, P., Kamat, A. M., . . . Pisters, L. L. (2007). Viable germ cell tumor at postchemotherapy retroperitoneal lymph node dissection: can we predict patients at risk of disease progression? *Cancer, 110*(12), 2700-2708.

Stephenson, A. J., Bosl, G. J., Motzer, R. J., Kattan, M. W., Stasi, J., Bajorin, D. F., & Sheinfeld, J. (2005). Retroperitoneal lymph node dissection for nonseminomatous germ cell testicular cancer: impact of patient selection factors on outcome. *J Clin Oncol, 23*(12), 2781-2788.

Steyerberg, E. W., Donohue, J. P., Gerl, A., Toner, G. C., Schraffordt Koops, H., Fossa, S. D., & Keizer, H. J. (1997). Residual masses after chemotherapy for metastatic testicular cancer: the clinical implications of the association between retroperitoneal and pulmonary histology. Re-analysis of Histology in Testicular Cancer (ReHiT) Study Group. *J Urol, 158*(2), 474-478.

Svatek, R. S., Spiess, P. E., Sundi, D., Tu, S. M., Tannir, N. M., Brown, G. A., . . . Pisters, L. L. (2009). Long-term outcome for men with teratoma found at postchemotherapy retroperitoneal lymph node dissection. *Cancer, 115*(6), 1310-1317.

Tognoni, P. G., Foster, R. S., McGraw, P., Heilman, D., Bihrle, R., Rowland, R. G., . . . Donohue, J. P. (1998). Combined post-chemotherapy retroperitoneal lymph node dissection and resection of chest tumor under the same anesthetic is appropriate based on morbidity and tumor pathology. *J Urol, 159*(6), 1833-1835.

Toner, G. C., Panicek, D. M., Heelan, R. T., Geller, N. L., Lin, S. Y., Bajorin, D., . . . et al. (1990). Adjunctive surgery after chemotherapy for nonseminomatous germ cell tumors: recommendations for patient selection. *J Clin Oncol, 8*(10), 1683-1694.

Vergouwe, Y., Steyerberg, E. W., Eijkemans, M. J., Albers, P., & Habbema, J. D. (2003). Predictors of occult metastasis in clinical stage I nonseminoma: a systematic review. *J Clin Oncol, 21*(22), 4092-4099.

Vugrin, D., Whitmore, W. F., Jr., Herr, H., Sogani, P., & Golbey, R. B. (1982). Adjuvant vinblastine, actinomycin D, bleomycin, cyclophosphamide and cis-platinum chemotherapy regimen with and without maintenance in patients with resected stage IIB testis cancer. *J Urol, 128*(4), 715-717.

Weissbach, L., & Hartlapp, J. H. (1991). Adjuvant chemotherapy of metastatic stage II nonseminomatous testis tumor. *J Urol, 146*(5), 1295-1298.

Westermann, D. H., Schefer, H., Thalmann, G. N., Karamitopoulou-Diamantis, E., Fey, M. F., & Studer, U. E. (2008). Long-term followup results of 1 cycle of adjuvant bleomycin, etoposide and cisplatin chemotherapy for high risk clinical stage I nonseminomatous germ cell tumors of the testis. *J Urol, 179*(1), 163-166.

Williams, S. D., Stablein, D. M., Einhorn, L. H., Muggia, F. M., Weiss, R. B., Donohue, J. P., . . . et al. (1987). Immediate adjuvant chemotherapy versus observation with treatment at relapse in pathological stage II testicular cancer. *N Engl J Med, 317*(23), 1433-1438. doi: 10.1056/NEJM198712033172303

Wood, D. P., Jr., Herr, H. W., Heller, G., Vlamis, V., Sogani, P. C., Motzer, R. J., . . . Sullivan, L. D. (1992). Distribution of retroperitoneal metastases after chemotherapy in patients with nonseminomatous germ cell tumors. *J Urol, 148*(6), 1812-1815; discussion 1815-1816.

Wood, D. P., Jr., Herr, H. W., Motzer, R. J., Reuter, V., Sogani, P. C., Morse, M. J., & Bosl, G. J. (1992). Surgical resection of solitary metastases after chemotherapy in patients with nonseminomatous germ cell tumors and elevated serum tumor markers. *Cancer, 70*(9), 2354-2357.

Wood, L., Kollmannsberger, C., Jewett, M., Chung, P., Hotte, S., O'Malley, M., . . . Warde, P. (2010). Canadian consensus guidelines for the management of testicular germ cell cancer. *Can Urol Assoc J, 4*(2), e19-38.

Xiao, H., Mazumdar, M., Bajorin, D. F., Sarosdy, M., Vlamis, V., Spicer, J., . . . Motzer, R. J. (1997). Long-term follow-up of patients with good-risk germ cell tumors treated with etoposide and cisplatin. *J Clin Oncol, 15*(7), 2553-2558.

3

Diagnostic Imaging of Intracranial Germ Cell Tumors: A Review

Takamitsu Fujimaki
Department of Neurosurgery,
Saitama Medical University, Moroyama,
Japan

1. Introduction

Intracranial germ cell tumors (CNS GCTs) are malignant neoplasms affecting mostly children and young adults. About 95% of affected patients are less than 24 years of age (Figure 1) [1], and males are affected more often than females, approximately three-quarters to four-fifths of patients being male [1, 2].

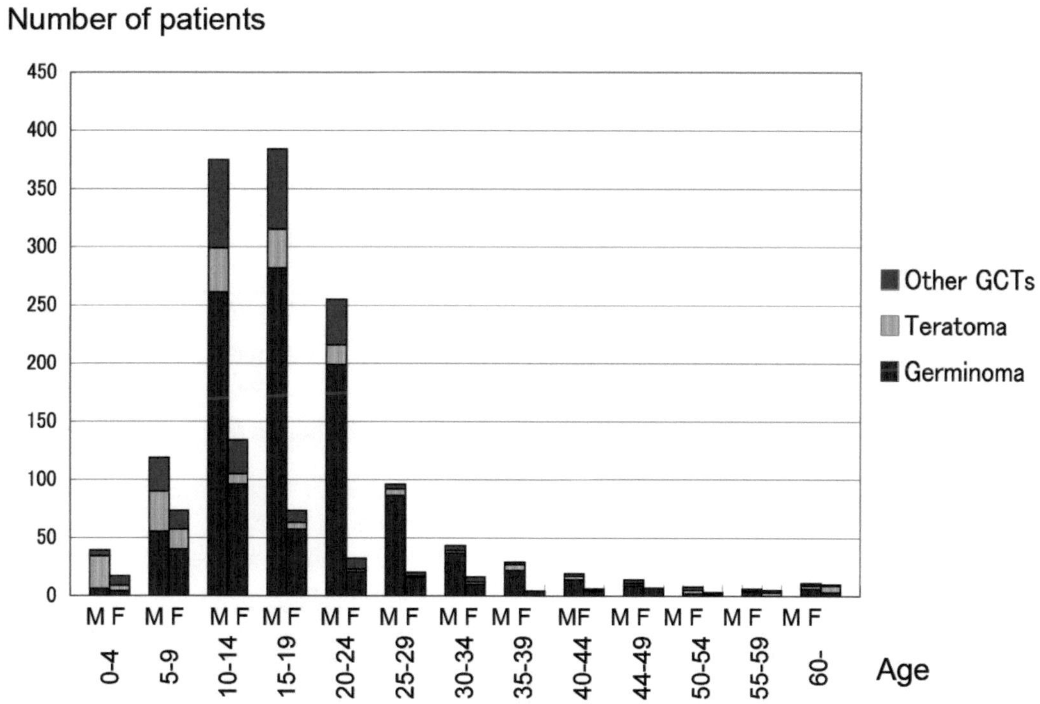

Fig. 1. Age and sex distribution of germ cell tumors (The Brain Tumor Registry of Japan (1)).

CNS GCTs are histologically classified into several histological subtypes, i.e. germinoma, teratoma (mature teratoma, immature teratoma, teratoma with malignant transformation), embryonal carcinoma, yolk sac tumor and choriocarcinoma [3, 4], and some are composed of a mixture of these subtypes. Germinomas are the most frequent histological subtype, followed in order by teratomas, choriocarcinomas, embryonal carcinomas and yolk sac tumors. Mixtures of these tumors are also common, and in fact one third of intracranial germ cell tumors are of mixed types. Among these, germinomas show typical histological patterns, being similar to dysgerminoma of the ovary or seminoma of the testis. They are composed of large round cells and small lymphocytes, thus their histological feature is known as the "two cell pattern".

The most frequently affected site is the pineal gland, followed by the neurohyphophyseal (or "suprasellar") region (Figure 2). However, these tumors can also arise in the basal ganglia or any other intracranial location.

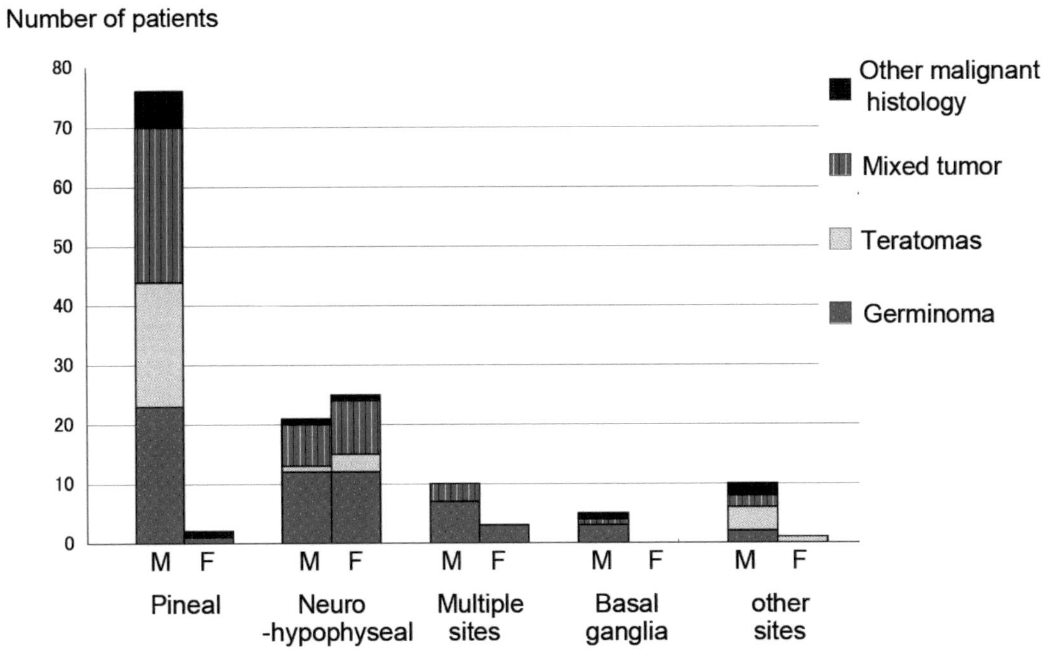

Fig. 2. Location and distribution of histological subtypes (according to Matsutani et al. (2)).

Although, biologically, all intracranial germ cell tumors, except for mature teratomas, are malignant, their clinical characteristics differ. Germinomas respond well to chemo-radiotherapy and their prognosis is relatively good. Mixed tumors composed of any type of teratoma and germinoma are also responsive to appropriate forms of combined therapy including surgery, radiation and/or chemotherapy, and thus their prognosis is better than that of other histological subtypes such as embryonal carcinoma, yolk sac tumor, choriocarcinoma or their mixtures (the so-called "poor prognosis" group), which require more intensive forms of chemo-radiotherapy [5, 6]. For this reason, accurate differential diagnosis of these histological subtypes is very important in a clinical setting.

2. Modalities important for diagnosis of CNS GCTs

Although pathological diagnosis by biopsy is essential for the planning of appropriate treatment for CNS GCTs, tentative histological diagnosis also plays a significant role in deciding the optimal surgical strategy. In this connection, both neuroimaging and assessment of tumor markers are important. Some CNS GCTs produce tumor markers that are helpful for indicating the histological subtype (Table 1). Typically, choriocarcinoma produces the beta-subunit of human chorionic gonadotropin (β-hCG) whereas yolk sac tumor produces alpha-fetoprotein (α-FP). If the serum level of β-hCG alone is elevated to more than 500 mIU/ml, or if that of α-FP alone is elevated to more than 500 ng/mL, then pure choriocarcinoma or yolk sac tumor is considered highly likely, respectively. The levels of markers associated with mixed germ cell tumors may vary according to the histological elements present. These tumor markers, together with the neuroimaging features discussed later, allow the histological subtypes of CNS GCTs to be assessed before surgery. As is the case for other CNS neoplasms, etiologic factors such as tumor location and patient age are also helpful for accurate diagnosis. As mentioned previously, the pineal gland is one of the most frequent sites for CNS GCTs. If a tumor is found in the pineal region in a teenage boy, it is highly likely to be a CNS GCT. Other tumors can arise in this region, but at a lower frequency in this age group. More detailed diagnosis should be made on the basis of neuroimaging features, together with tumor markers.

	β-hCG	α-FP
Germinoma	— ~ ↑	—
Mature teratoma	—	—
Immature teratoma Teratoma with malignant transformation	—	— ~ ↑
Embyronal carcinoma	—	— ~ ↑
Yolk sac tumor	—	↑↑↑
Choriocarcinoma	↑↑↑	—

Table 1. Tumor markers and histological subtypes

2.1 MRI and CT features of CNS GCTs

2.1.1 Pineal tumors

For tumors in the pineal gland in children or young adults, differential diagnoses are limited. Although many CNS tumors can occur in this location, those that apparently arise within the pineal gland itself are limited. Many tumors, such as meningiomas, gliomas or ependymomas, can occur in the pineal region, but they extend from neighboring structures and do not arise in the pineal gland itself. Most pineal tumors in the true sense are CNS GCTs or pineal parenchymal tumors, i.e. pineocytoma, pineal parenchymal tumor of intermediate differentiation, or pineoblastoma. All of these tumors can cause obstructive hydrocephalus due to compression to the aqueduct. Thus, the initial symptoms and neuroimaging finding of pineal CNS GCTs often reflect increased intracranial pressure due to hydrocephalus (Figure 3).

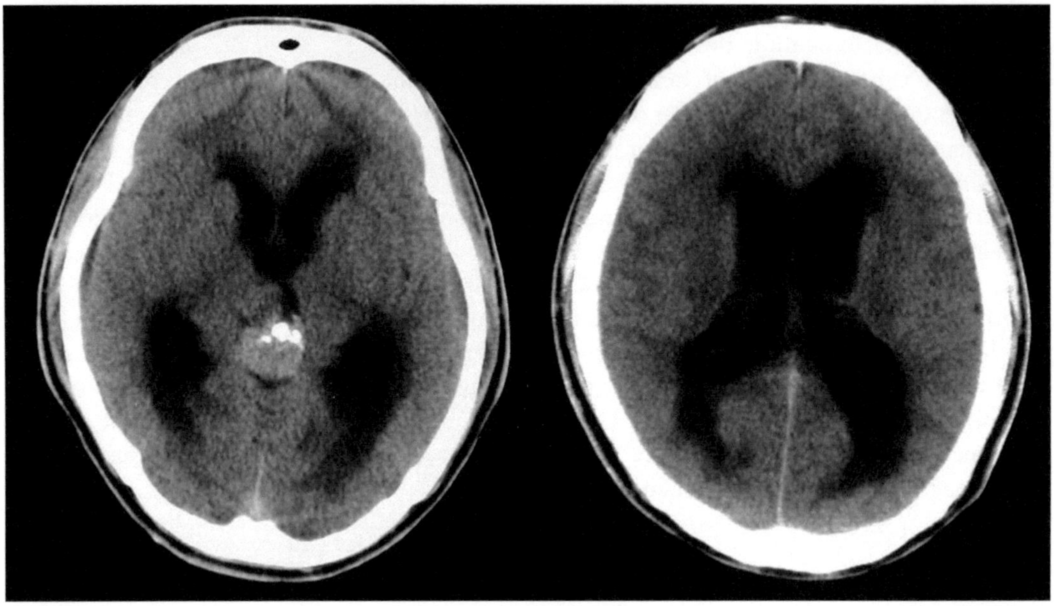

Fig. 3. Computed tomography (CT) scans of a pineal germinoma on admission. Marked hydrocephalus is evident together with the pineal mass.

Among CNS GCTs, germinomas and teratomas each show a peculiar pattern. Germinomas show slightly high to high density on plain (non-enhanced) CT scans. The border is clear where the tumor faces the cerebrospinal fluid space (cistern or ventricle), but somewhat obscure where the tumor faces the brain parenchyma. These tumors show marked homogeneous enhancement with contrast media [7-9]. Small intratumoral cysts may be present [9], and calcifications within the tumor are frequently evident [10, 11]. On T1-weighted MRI (the most basic MRI scanning), they appear as a well demarcated mass with a slightly low signal intensity. On T2-weighted images (which is another basic MRI scanning and in which tissues containing more water molecules show high signal) the germinomas show slightly high intensity (Figure 4) [9, 12-14]. Teratomas appear as heterogeneous masses, since they contain many histological elements [9, 12, 14]. CT shows that they are well demarcated, containing multiple small and large cysts and some calcifications. The entire tumor, or some part of it, may be well enhanced [9]. Teratomas sometimes contain fatty tissue, which is well detected by MRI, showing high signal intensity on both T1- and T2-weighted images. If such fatty tissues are detected by MRI, the tumor is highly likely to be a teratoma, or at least to contain a teratomatous component [9, 14]. On MRI, teratomas are well enhanced with gadolinium, except for cystic components (Figure 5). As mentioned above, teratomas may be benign or contain immature elements or malignant components. When the tumor's growth rate is high, perifocal edema may be detected on T2-weighted images [15].

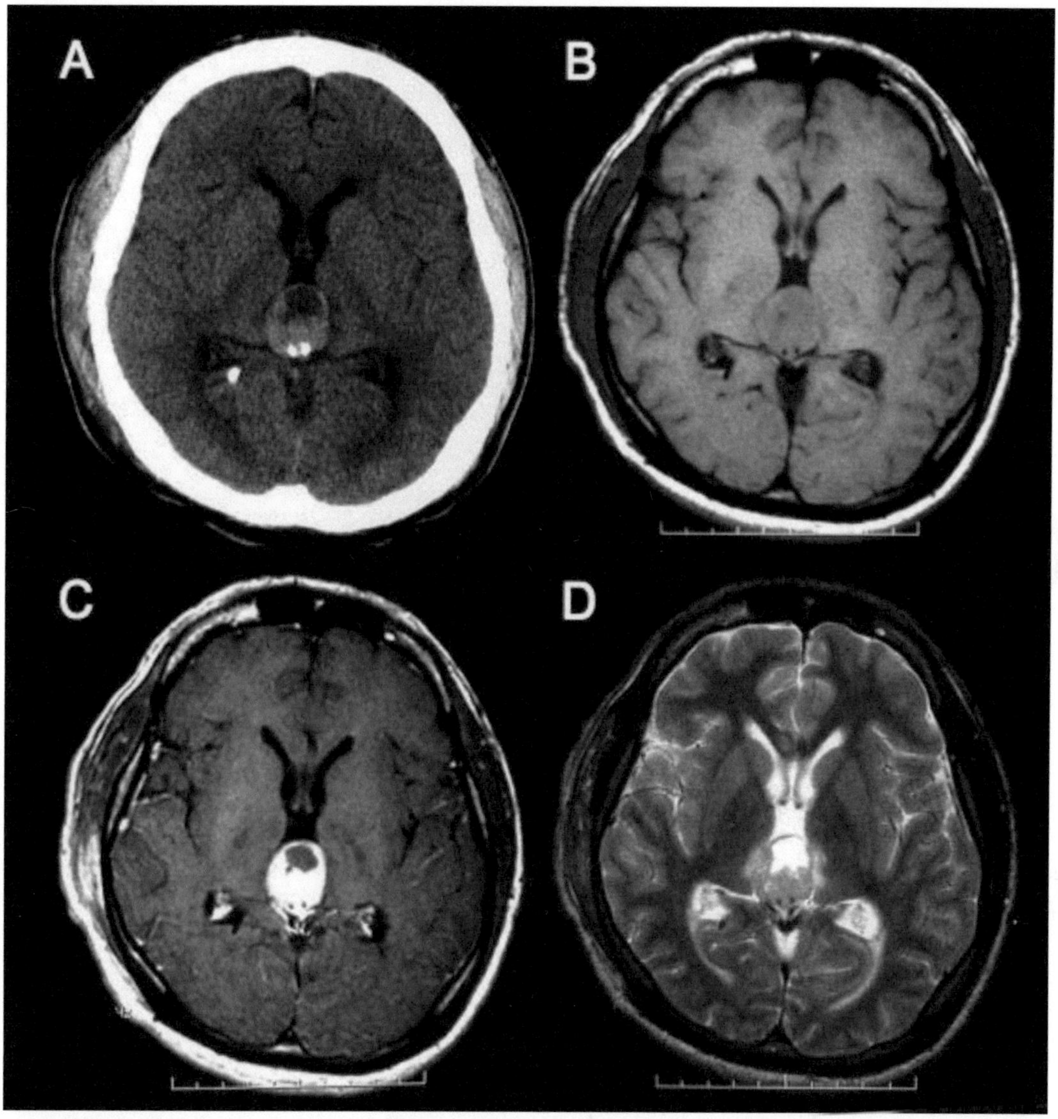

Fig. 4. Pineal germinoma in an 18-year-old boy. (A) CT scan shows a slightly high-density mass in the pineal region, together with a cyst and some calcifications. A ventricular drainage tube is inserted into the posterior horn of the right lateral ventricle. The tumor shows slightly low signal intensity on the T1-weighted image (B) and slightly high signal intensity on the T2-weighted image (D). The tumor is homogeneously well enhanced by gadolinium (C).

Other malignant subtypes are difficult to diagnose on the basis of neuroimaging features alone, but certain tendencies are evident for some tumors; yolk sac tumors tend to be irregular in shape, and unlike germimonas, show isodensity or slightly low density by non-enhanced CT [9]. Occasionally, the onset of choriocarcinoma may be accompanied by intracranial bleeding (Figure 6). In young adult or pediatric patients presenting with intraventricular hemorrhage, the possible presence of occult choriocarcinoma other than cerebrovascular conditions such as arteriovenous malformation should be considered. As mentioned above, measurement of the serum β-hCG level is helpful in this situation. These malignant subtypes or mixed germ cell tumors with these elements are more aggressive than germinomas or teratomas, and thus often also have perifocal edema.

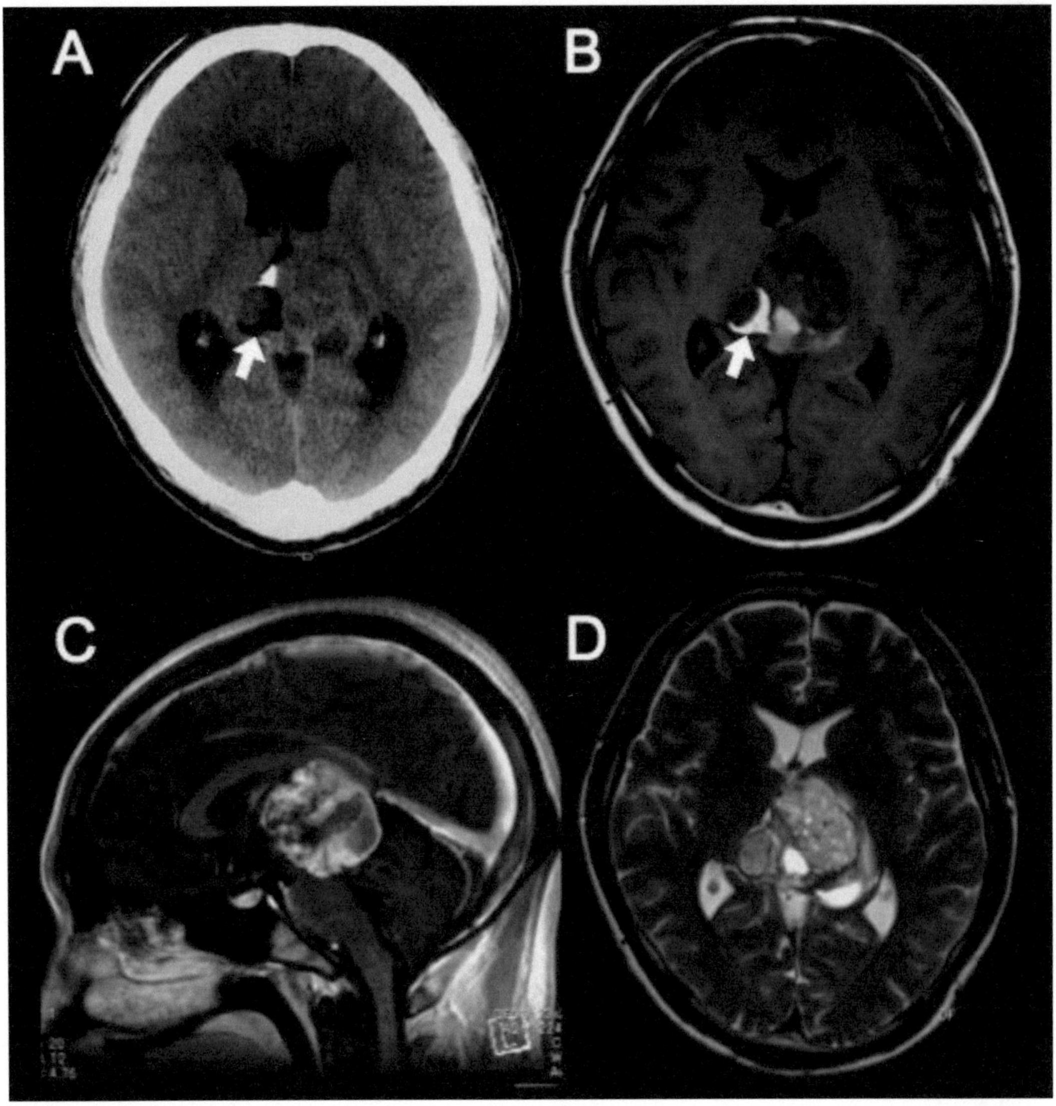

Fig. 5. Mixed germ cell tumor composed of immature teratoma and yolk sac tumor. The tumor contains calcification and fatty tissue. The low-density area evident on CT (white arrow, A) or the area of high signal intensity (white arrow, B) on the T1-weighted image indicates the presence of fatty tissue. The tumor is heterogeneously enhanced (C). The T2-weighted image also shows a heterogeneous pattern (D).

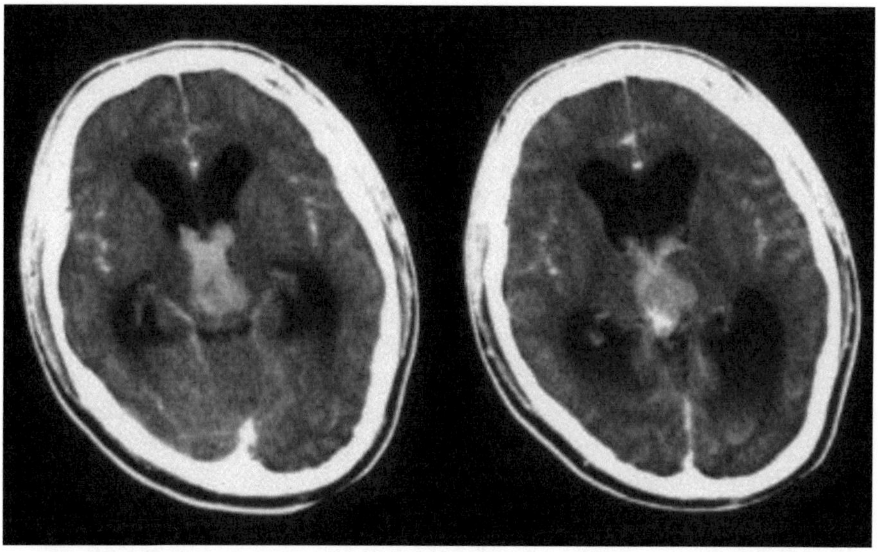

Fig. 6. A 16-year-old boy who was admitted in a comatose state. CT scans show intraventricular hemorrhage with hydrocephalus. The level of beta-hCG was markedly elevated. The diagnosis of choriocarcinoma was confirmed by biopsy three weeks later.

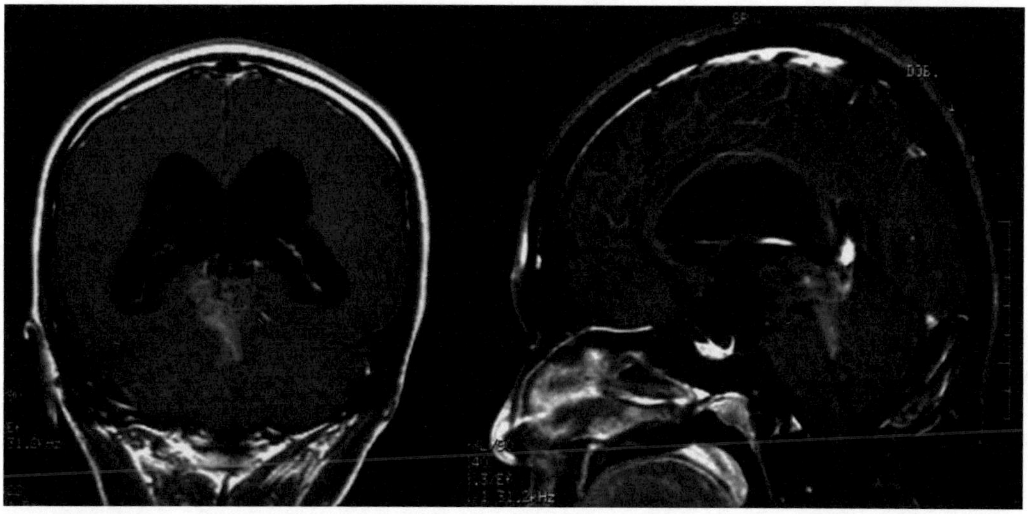

Fig. 7. A 26-year-old woman with a pineal parenchymal tumor showing intermediate differentiation. The tumor extends to the quadrigeminal and supracerebellar cisterns.

Pineal parenchymal tumors are rare, and reports on their neuroimaging features are limited. However, CT scan can often detect calcifications, and the pattern differs from that of germ cell tumors. Such calcifications correspond to an "exploded" pattern of preexisting pineal calcification, whereas those of germinomas are included within the tumor [10]. On MRI, differentiation between CNS GCTs and pineal parenchymal tumors is difficult [15]. For example, pineocytoma also shows slightly high signal intensity on T2-weighted images. However, pineoblastoma, the most malignant form of pineal parenchymal tumor, shows a signal that is iso-intense with gray matter on T2-weighted images, and invades into surrounding structures [15]; perifocal edema may also be present. If a tumor extends expansively to fill the quadrigeminal to supracerebellar cistern frontal to the cerebellar culmen, it may be a pineal parenchymal tumor rather than a germ cell tumor (Figure 7) [13, 15].

2.1.2 Tumors of the neurohypophyseal region

The neurohypophysis or suprasellar area is the second-most frequent site for CNS GSTs. The basic neuroimaging characteristics of CNS GSTs in this location are not different from those of pineal ones in terms of density or signal intensity, enhancement pattern, and so on (Figure 8). However, calcification demonstrated by CT is somewhat different, as there is no "preexisting pineal calcification" in this area. Other tumors such as pituitary adenoma and craniopharyngioma, or inflammatory diseases such as Langerhans cell histiocytosis (LCH), can arise here [16, 17]. Most CNS GCTs arise from the pituitary stalk or hypothalamic area, whereas pituitary adenomas occur within the pituitary gland itself. Moreover, pituitary adenomas are relatively rare in the pediatric population. For these reasons, there is generally no problem in recognizing pituitary adenomas. However, differentiation between CNS GCTs and some of the other tumors mentioned above is sometimes not so easy. Any tumor showing multiple cysts and calcifications in this area might be a teratoma or a craniopharyngioma [18]. However, teratomas arise more often in the pineal region than in the neurohypophysis. Matsutani et al. reported that among 153 CNS GCTs, only 4 teratomas arose in the neurohypophyseal region.[2]. The incidence of CNS GCTs in the pediatric population is 15% or less [1]. Thus the frequency of neurohypophyseal teratoma among all pediatric brain tumors might be around 0.4%. In contrast, the incidence of craniopharyngioma in the pediatric population is around 9% [1]. Thus a tumor with multiple cysts and calcifications is 20 times more likely to be a craniopharyngioma. Inflammatory diseases in this location, for example LCH, are sometimes difficult to differentiate from small CNS GCTs [19].

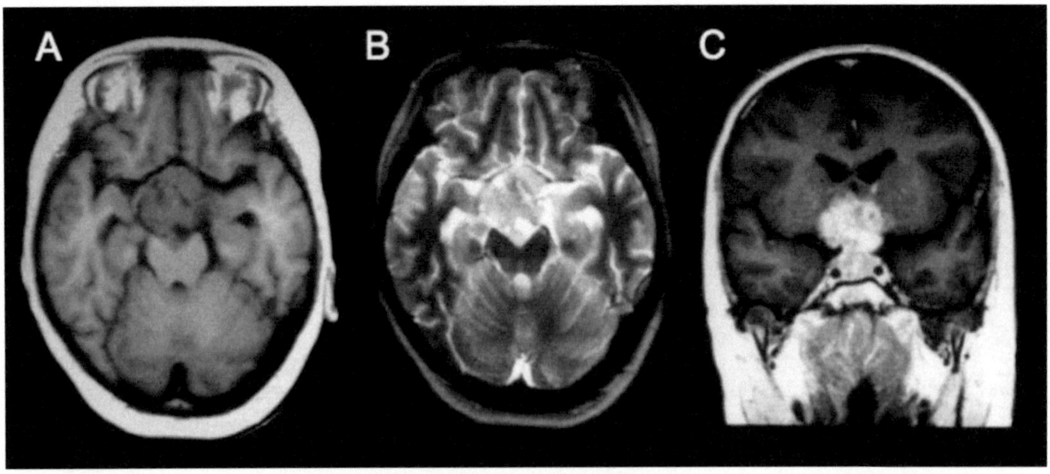

Fig. 8. Neurohypophyseal germinoma in a 12-year-old girl. A large tumor is evident in the basal cistern. The tumor shows slightly low signal intensity on the T1-weighted image (A) and slightly high signal intensity on the T2-weighted image (B). A coronal image after enhancement shows that the tumor is well enhanced.

Sometimes "bifocal" tumors arise in the neurohypophysis and pineal region (Figure 9). Most of these tumors are germinomas [20], but other histological subtypes of CNS GCT have also been reported [21]. As other central nervous system tumors rarely present this "bifocal" pattern, it is strongly suggestive of CNS GCT, especially germinoma.

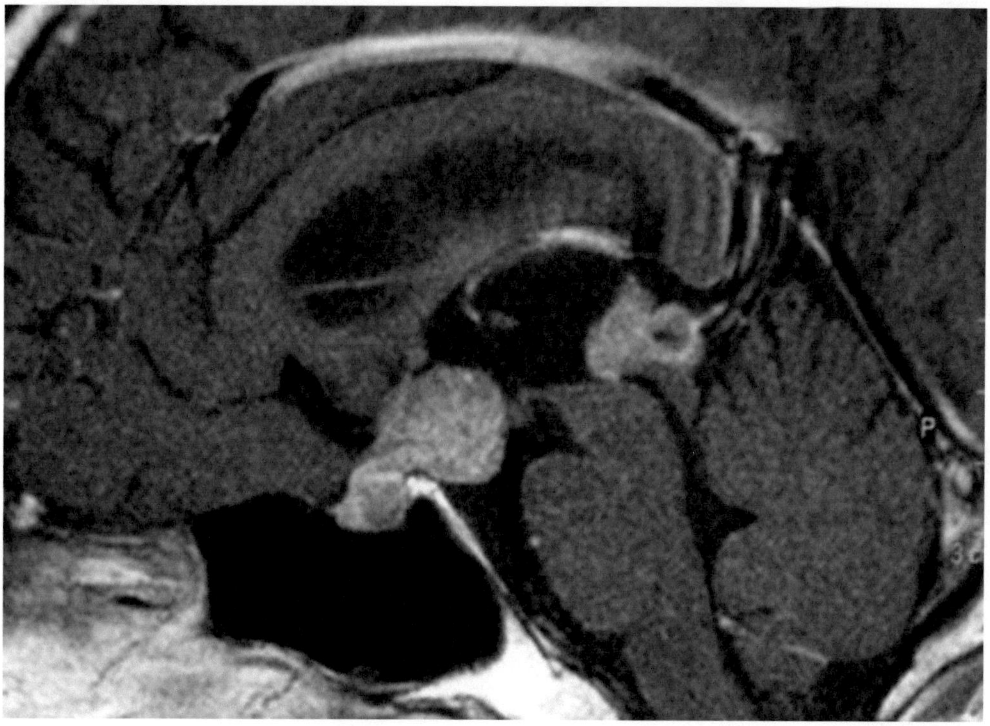

Fig. 9. A "bifocal" pattern germinoma is demonstrated on an enhanced sagittal image.

2.1.3 Other locations

Although CNS GCTs sometimes affect the basal ganglia, the neuroimaging features of GCTs in this location differ from those at other locations. Most CNS GCTs affecting the basal ganglia are germinomas, and are invasive. They show no mass effect or enhancement, initially [22-26]. Slightly high signal intensity on FLAIR or T2-weighted images is sometimes the only prominent finding. Thus, diagnosis at this stage is often difficult, and may be delayed even if a patient has undergone neuroimaging at an earlier stage. Later, the tumor may show exhibit a mass effect, enhancement, or even cysts. Tumor invasion to the pyramidal tract can cause hemiparesis. Hemiatrophy of the cerebral peduncle due to pyramidal tract impairment can be observed in patients with long-standing neurological symptoms (Figure 10) [24].

2.1.4 Spinal images

Occasionally, but not rarely, a tumor may show dissemination via the cerebrospinal fluid at initial presentation (Figure 11). Therefore, once a CNS GCT is suspected, enhanced MRI of the whole spine should be conducted.

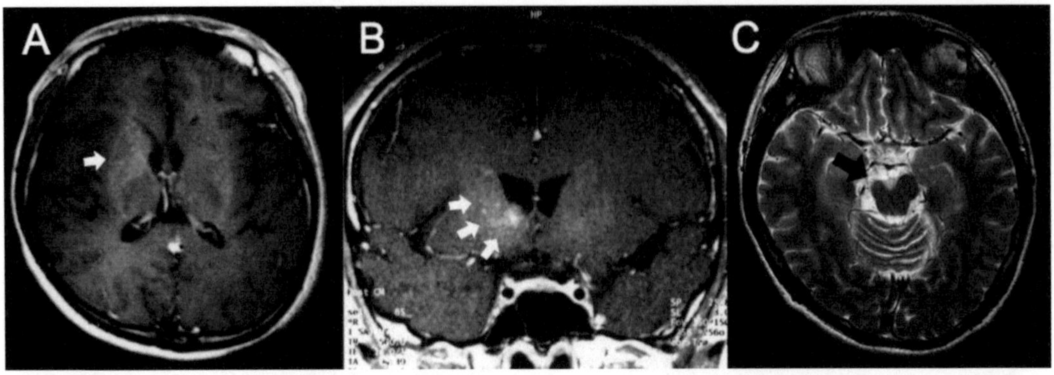

Fig. 10. Germinoma in the basal ganglia of a 21-year-old man. A gadolinium-enhanced MR image at initial presentation was diagnosed as normal, although the patient presented with slight left hemiparesis (A). Eight months later, enhanced MRI demonstrated slight enhancement (B), and biopsy confirmed the diagnosis of germinoma (B). The tumor was well controlled after chemo-radiotherapy, but the patient remained hemiparetic. Hemiatrophy of the cerebral peduncle was evident after 12 years (C).

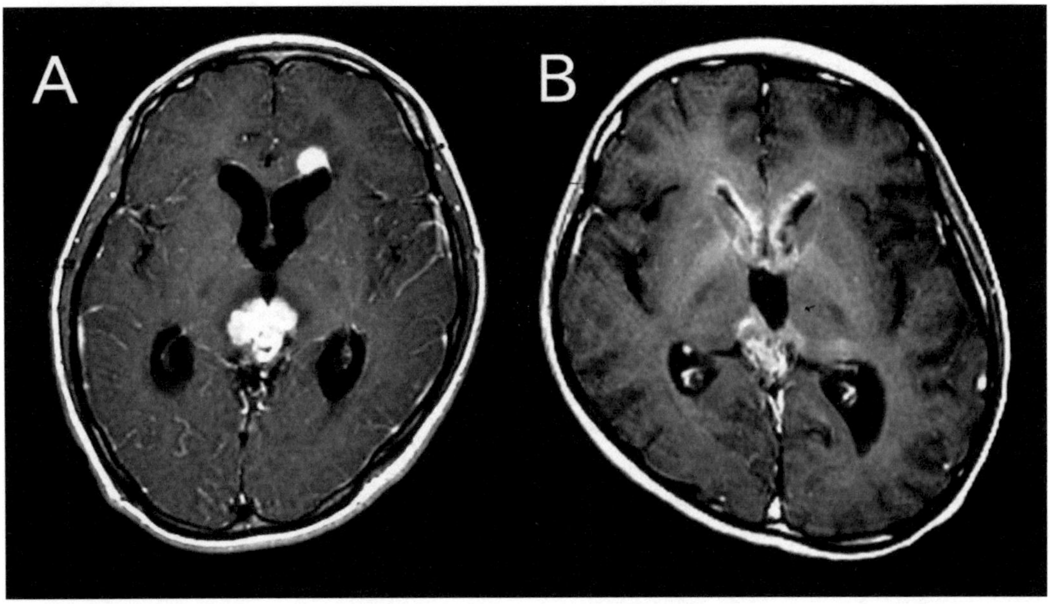

Fig. 11. MRI scans obtained at initial presentation, showing dissemination along the cerebrospinal fluid or subpial space in an 18-year-old boy (A) and a 13-year-old boy (B).

2.2 Other modalities for neuroimaging of CNS GCTs

Recently, more advanced techniques such as magnetic resonance spectroscopy (MRS) or positron emission tomography (PET) have been employed for diagnosing CNS diseases. Although reports on imaging of CNS GCTs using advanced techniques such as PET or MRS are limited, some have indicated the usefulness of these modalities for diagnosis or decision-making in a clinical setting. Increased tracer uptake has been demonstrated using both methionine-PET (MET-PET) and fluorodeoxyglucose-PET (FDG-PET) in patients with germinomas. However, FDG-PET does not demonstrate increased uptake in some germinomas [22, 27]. For invasive tumors in the basal ganglia, Kawai et al. reported that they were able to decide an appropriate biopsy point on the basis of MET-PET images when the exact location of the tumor was unclear in usual MRI or CT images.[23]

On the basis of a MRS study, Harris et al. described that CNS GCTs have a high lipid and macromolecule (LMM) concentration in comparison with other brain tumors. They also detected taurine in germinomas and pineal parenchymal tumors [28]. Although at a preliminary stage of evaluation, MRS seems to be an interesting modality for diagnosis of CNS GCTS.

3. Conclusion

Through detailed interpretation of neuroimaging findings, together with tumor markers and other demographic clinical information, it is possible to determine the histological subtypes of CNS GCTs. With advanced imaging techniques, further improvement of diagnostic accuracy may be achievable, together with better understanding of the detailed biological characteristics of CNS GCTs.

4. References

[1] The Committee of the Brain Tumor Registry of Japan, Report of Brain Tumor Registry of Japan (1984-2000), 12th Edition. Neurol Med Chir (Tokyo), 2009. 49(supplement).
[2] Matsutani, M., et al., Primary intracranial germ cell tumors: a clinical analysis of 153 histologically verified cases. J Neurosurg, 1997. 86(3): p. 446-55.
[3] The International Agency for Research on Cancer, WHO Classification of Tumours of the Central Nervous System, 4th ed., D.N. Louis, et al., Editors. 2007, IARC: Lyon.
[4] Fujimaki, T., Central nervous system germ cell tumors: classification, clinical features, and treatment with a historical overview. J Child Neurol, 2009. 24(11): p. 1439-45.
[5] Matsutani, M., Combined chemotherapy and radiation therapy for CNS germ cell tumors--the Japanese experience. J Neurooncol, 2001. 54(3): p. 311-6.
[6] Kanamori, M., et al., Optimal treatment strategy for intracranial germ cell tumors: a single institution analysis. J Neurosurg Pediatr, 2009. 4(6): p. 506-14.
[7] Chang, T., et al., CT of pineal tumors and intracranial germ-cell tumors. Am J Roentgenol, 1989. 153(6): p. 1269-74.
[8] Salzman, K.L., et al., Primary intracranial germ cell tumors: clinicopathologic review of 32 cases. Pediatr Pathol Lab Med, 1997. 17(5): p. 713-27.
[9] Fujimaki, T., et al., CT and MRI features of intracranial germ cell tumors. J Neurooncol, 1994. 19(3): p. 217-26.
[10] Smirniotopoulos, J.G., E.J. Rushing, and H. Mena, Pineal region masses: differential diagnosis. Radiographics, 1992. 12(3): p. 577-96.
[11] Packer, R.J., B.H. Cohen, and K. Cooney, Intracranial germ cell tumors. Oncologist, 2000. 5(4): p. 312-20.
[12] Sumida, M., et al., MRI of intracranial germ cell tumours. Neuroradiology, 1995. 37(1): p. 32-7.

[13] Fujimaki, T., Central Nervous System Germ Cell Tumor, in Tumors of the Central Nervous System Volume 4, Brain Tumors (Part 2), M.A. Hayat, Editor. 2011, Springer: Dordrecht. p. 71-77.
[14] Zee, C.S., et al., MR imaging of pineal region neoplasms. J Comput Assist Tomogr, 1991. 15(1): p. 56-63.
[15] Korogi, Y., M. Takahashi, and Y. Ushio, MRI of pineal region tumors. J Neurooncol, 2001. 54(3): p. 251-61.
[16] Isoo, A., et al., Langerhans cell histiocytosis limited to the pituitary-hypothalamic axis--two case reports. Neurol Med Chir (Tokyo), 2000. 40(10): p. 532-5.
[17] Kaltsas, G.A., et al., Hypothalamo-pituitary abnormalities in adult patients with Langerhans cell histiocytosis: clinical, endocrinological, and radiological features and response to treatment. J Clin Endocrinol Metab, 2000. 85(4): p. 1370-6.
[18] Donovan, J.L. and G.M. Nesbit, Distinction of masses involving the sella and suprasellar space: specificity of imaging features. Am J Roentgenol, 1996. 167(3): p. 597-603.
[19] Prayer, D., et al., MR imaging presentation of intracranial disease associated with Langerhans cell histiocytosis. Am J Neuroradiol, 2004. 25(5): p. 880-91.
[20] Sugiyama, K., et al., Intracranial germ-cell tumor with synchronous lesions in the pineal and suprasellar regions: report of six cases and review of the literature. Surg Neurol, 1992. 38(2): p. 114-20.
[21] Cuccia, V. and D. Alderete, Suprasellar/pineal bifocal germ cell tumors. Childs Nerv Syst, 2010. 26(8): p. 1043-9.
[22] Phi, J.H., et al., Germinomas in the basal ganglia: magnetic resonance imaging classification and the prognosis. J Neurooncol, 2010. 99(2): p. 227-36.
[23] Kawai, N., et al., Targeting optimal biopsy location in basal ganglia germinoma using (11)C-methionine positron emission tomography. Surg Neurol, 2008. 70(4): p. 408-13; discussion 413.
[24] Ozelame, R.V., et al., Basal ganglia germinoma in children with associated ipsilateral cerebral and brainstem hemiatrophy. Pediatr Radiol, 2006. 36(4): p. 325-30.
[25] Takano, T., et al., Sequential MRI findings in a patient with a germ cell tumor in the basal ganglia. Brain Dev, 1993. 15(4): p. 283-7.
[26] Higano, S., et al., Germinoma originating in the basal ganglia and thalamus: MR and CT evaluation. Am J Neuroradiol, 1994. 15(8): p. 1435-41.
[27] Kelly, P.A., et al., Positron emission tomography in the diagnosis and management of intracranial germ cell tumours. Horm Res, 2009. 72(3): p. 190-6.
[28] Harris, L.M., et al., Short echo time single voxel 1H magnetic resonance spectroscopy in the diagnosis and characterisation of pineal tumours in children. Pediatr Blood Cancer, 2011. 57(6): p. 972-7.

4

Testicular Germ Cell Tumours – A European and UK Perspective

Nikhil Vasdev and Andrew C. Thorpe
Department of Urology
Freeman Hospital
Newcastle upon Tyne
United Kingdom

1. Introduction

Testicular Germ Cell tumours (TGCTs) account for between 1% and 1.5% of male neoplasms and 5% of urological tumours in general, with 3-10 new cases occurring per 100,000 males/per year in Western society (1-3). Testicular germ cell tumours (TGCTs) are the most frequent solid tumour of Caucasian adolescents and young adult males and are a diverse group of neoplasms that can also present in extragonadal sites. Within Europe, there has been a general increase in the incidence of TGCTs noted initially in the 1970s and 1980s (4). Over recent years the incidence of TGCTs has risen markedly, making it imperative to understand how and why these tumours arise.

In this book chapter we present the incidence and clinical presentation, classification, epidemiology and aetiology, molecular developments, tumour markers, staging, management strategies including the role of chemotherapy, radiotherapy and Reteroperitoneal lymph node dissection (RPLND) and follow up protocol followed in the United Kingdom (UK) and Europe as per the 2011 European Association of Urology (EAU) guidelines.

2. Incidence and clinical presentation

Testicular Germ Cell tumours (TGCTs) are broadly divided into Seminomas, which resemble primordial germ cells (PGCs) and Non-Seminoma, which are either undifferentiated (embryonal carcinoma) or differentiated (exhibiting a degree of embryonic (teratoma) or extra-embryonic (yolk sac choriocarcinoma) pattern (5). The commonest age range of presentation of TGCTs is between 20-45 years. Patients rarely tend to be younger than 15 years or older than 60 years. Based on the type of TGSTs, Seminomas typically arise later in life, with a mean age at presentation of 35 years of age compared with 25 years of age for non-seminomas. Although these morphologies and differences in age at presentation could suggest underlying differences between seminomas and non-seminomas, several lines of evidence support a common underlying pathogenesis. Approximately 15% of TGCTs are mixed tumours that contain both seminoma and non-seminoma elements (6).

The commonest presentation of TGCTs is a painless unilateral mass in the scrotum when the patient feels the mass itself. In other situations the patient has an incidental mass diagnosed when presenting with other symptoms of a concomitant testicular pathology such as epididymitits. It is interesting to note that 10% of patients presenting with epididymitis present can present with a TGCTs (1, 2). Another common symptom of presentation is testicular pain (1) seen in up to 20% of patient with TGCTs. In certain cases up to 27% of patients have local pain which could be attributed to a degree of local invasion (1). Up to 1-2% of TGCTs present bilaterally. Paraneoplastic symptoms such as gynaecomastia can be seen in up to 7% of patients at initial presentation. Additional symptoms include lower back pain and loin pain (1, 2).

When a patient presents with a testicular mass it is extremely important to elicit a detailed history which includes duration of symptoms, whether the mass is painful or painless, change in size of mass, sexual history, concomitant lower urinary tract symptoms, previous history of surgery, infertility or mumps and family history of testicular cancer. There is evidence to suggest that delay in presentation is more of a problem than delay in referral and this has prompted some authors to suggest that a public education campaign might be helpful (7,8).

The radiological investigation of choice for testicular cancer is an ultrasound throughout Europe. The main advantage lies with the fact that an ultrasound is non radiation exposure scan and is relatively inexpensive. The current sensitivity and specificity of an ultrasound of testis is 100% (9). In patients with an equivocal diagnosis a Magnetic resonance imaging (MRI) offers a sensitivity of 100% and a specificity of 95-100% (10), but its high cost does not justify its use for diagnosis.

3. Classification

As the 2011 European Association of Urology (EAU) guidelines testicular cancer is classified according to the 2004 World health organization (WHO) guidelines (11). From the perspective of this book chapter we will confine our discussion to Testicular Germ Cell Tumours only.

1. Germ cell tumours
   - Intratubular germ cell neoplasia, unclassified type (IGCNU)
   - Seminoma (including cases with syncytiotrophoblastic cells)
   - Spermatocytic seminoma (mention if there is sarcomatous component)
   - Embryonal carcinoma
   - Yolk sac tumour
   - Choriocarcinoma
   - Teratoma (mature, immature, with malignant component)
   - Tumours with more than one histological type (specify percentage of individual components)
2. Sex cord/gonadal stromal tumours
   - Leydig cell tumour
   - Malignant Leydig cell tumour
   - Sertoli cell tumour
     - lipid-rich variant
     - sclerosing
     - large cell calcifying

- Malignant Sertoli cell tumour
- Granulosa cell tumour
  - adult type
  - juvenile type
- Thecoma/fibroma group of tumours
- Other sex cord/gonadal stromal tumours
  - incompletely differentiated
  - mixed
- Tumours containing germ cell and sex cord/gonadal stromal (gonadoblastoma)

3. Miscellaneous non-specific stromal tumours
   - Ovarian epithelial tumours
   - Tumours of the collecting ducts and rete testis
   - Tumours (benign and malignant) of non-specific stroma.

4. Epidemiology and aetiology

The Epidemiology and Aetiology of TGCTs has evolved over the past two decades.

4.1 Age

In the paediatric population i.e., patients ≤ 16 years, the commonest form of Testicular Tumours are Mature teratomas, rhabdomyosarcoma, epidermoid cyst, yolk sac and germ cell tumours. The commonest age group of patients affected with TGCTs is between 20-45 years. Teratomas are common between the age of 20-35 years while seminomas are more common between the ages of 25-45 years. In men above the age of 60 years the commonest tumour is a lymphoma.

4.2 Cryptorchidism

When patients present with cryptorchidism, there is risk of development of testicular tumour on both the effected side and contralateral side in the long term. The risk of TGCT in the Undescended Testis (UDT) is increased by 4 - 13 , with up to 7-10% of Testicular Cancers developing in UDT (12). There is a 5-10% risk of developing testicular cancer in the contralateral testis in those with a history of UDT (13). Premalignant changes within the UDT commence by the age of 3 years. However, an early orchidopexy does not completely eliminate the risk of developing testicular cancer in the long term.

4.3 Intratubular Germ Cell Neoplasia (IGCNU)

Intratubular germ cell neoplasia (IGCNU) is also known as carcinoma *in situ* (CIS) of the testis. The incidence of IGCNU in the overall population is 0.9%. Intratubular germ cell neoplasia is defined as a pre-invasive testicular germ cell lesion and is now believed an important precursor of TGCTs. The only TGCT not associated with IGCNU is a spermatocytic seminoma. When IGNU is present, the probability of progression to TGCTs increases by 50% over a duration of 5 years. At 7 years, the cumulative probability of developing a TGCTs increased to 70% (14).

The incidence of IGCNU is the contralateral testis in patients with TGCTs is 5-9%. The incidence however rises to 34% when the primary TGCTs has been diagnosed before the age of 40 years and the testicular volume is less than 12 ml. In both the above mentioned scenarios , the EAU guidelines recommends a biopsy of the contralateral testis. It is important to note that the presence of IGCNU in the ipsilateral testis does not have any bearing on the patients overall prognosis. Risk factors for IGCNU include cryptorchidism (UDT), extra-gonadal germ cell tumour, previous or contralateral TGCT (5%), atrophic testicle with a volume of less than 12 ml, early age of diagnosis of TGCTs i.e., ≤ 40 years, 45XO karyotype, Klinefelter's syndrome and infertility. Once IGCNU is diagnosed, local radiotherapy is the treatment of choice in solitary testis. Because this may produce infertility, the patient must be carefully counselled before treatment commences.

4.4 Maternal oestrogen exposure

Maternal Oestrogen Exposure (MOE) increases during pregnancy and hence increases the risk of crytorchidism and TGCT in the male offspring. The MOE with diethylstilboestrol increases the risk of TGCTs by a relative risk of 2.8 - 5.3% (13).

4.5 Subfertility

A history of subfertility and poor quality semen analysis increases the risk of testicular cancer by upto 1.6 times and from the Surveillance Epidemiology and End Results database by 20 times (14) .

4.6 Family history

Familial history of testicular tumours among first-grade relatives (father/brothers) has been associated with isochromosome of the short arm of chromosome 12 – i(12p) (15).

4.7 Additional factors

Additional factors such as tallness, previous history of Marijuana exposure, vasectomy, trauma, mumps and Human Immunodeficiency Virus (HIV) infection continue to be evaluated (13-15).

5. Genetic and cellular markers

Current research has indentified deregulation in the pluripotent programme of fetal germ cells (identified by specific markers such as M2A, C-KIT and OCT4/NANOG) is probably responsible for the development of IGCNU and germ cell neoplasia. There is overlap in the development to seminoma and embryonal carcinoma as shown by genomewide expression analysis and detection of alpha-fetoprotein (AFP) mRNA in some atypical seminoma (16,17).Continued genome wide screening studies and gene expression analysis data suggest testis cancer specific gene mutations on chromosomes 4, 5, 6 and 12 (namely expressing SPRY4, kit-Ligand and Synaptopodin) (18-20). Intratubular germ cell neoplasia shows alterations in the p53 in upto 66% of cases.

Newer developments continue to be made with regards to further molecular profiling of TGCTs. The current molecular developments include characterization of newer markers such as MAGEC2 expression. This newer marker allows a reliable distinction of seminoma from embryonal carcinomas. Therefore, MAGEC2 represents an additional tool for the differential diagnosis of testicular germ cell tumours (21).

6. Serum markers for TGCTs

For the successful management of TGCTs it is crucial to understand the molecular details, half lives and clinical applications of testicular tumour markers. In clinical practice with Europe and the UK, the three common tumour markers used include Alpha-fetoprotein (AFP), β- human chorionic gonadotrophin (β-HCG) and lactate dehydrogenase (LDH). All testicular tumour markers contribute to the patients diagnosis and more importantly to the final prognosis. When a patient is diagnosed with a TGCTs, tumour markers will be elevated in 51% of cases (22).

Alpha-fetoprotein (AFP) is expressed by trophoblastic elements within 50-70% of non-seminomatous germ cell tumour (NSGCT) and yolk sac tumours. In patients with an elevated AFP with Seminoma alone, this raises the suspicion of the presence of Non-seminomatous elements. The half life of AFP is 5-7 days and the normal serum levels are <10 ng/ml. β- human chorionic gonadotrophin (β-HCG) is produced by syntiotrophoblast elements. In patients with choriocarcinomas , β-HCG is elevated in 100% of cases. From the perspective of other TGCTs, β-HCG is elevated in 40% of cases of NSGCT and 10% of Seminomas. The half life of β-HCG is 24-36 hours and normal serum levels are < 5mIU/ml. About 90% of non-seminomatous tumours present with a rise in one or two of the markers.

Lactate dehydrogenase (LDH) is a less specific marker and is an ubiquitous enzyme elevated in serum from various causes, therefore is less specific. It is elevated in 10-20% of seminomas but may be elevated in 80% of patients with advanced testicular cancer (23). Other markers studied include Placental alkaline phosphatase (PLAP), which may be of value in monitoring patients with pure seminoma. placental alkaline phosphatase (PLAP) is a foetal enzyme and may be falsely elevated in smokers. Cytogenetic and molecular markers are available in specific centres, but at present only contribute to research studies. Measurement of serum AFP, hCG and LDH is mandatory, while that of PLAP is optional.

Testicular tumour serum markers are normally measured when a patient presents with a TGCT clinically. In Europe the Testicular tumour markers are measured 1-2 weeks following radical orchidectomy. The testicular tumour markers play an important role in assessing response to treatment and follow up. The presence of normal testicular tumour markers prior to orchidectomy does not normally exclude the presence of micrometastatic disease. However, the persistence of testicular tumour markers following post radical inguinal orchidectomy may occur in patients with hepatic dysfunction, hypogonadotropism and most importantly in metastatic disease.

It is also important to note that other malignancies may cause an elevation of testicular tumour markers. Liver, pancreatic, gastric and lung malignancies may cause an elevated AFP level. Pancreatic, liver, gastic, lung, breast, kidney and bladder cancer may cause an elevated β-HCG level. Prior to commencing chemotherapy all tumour markers must be performed to classify patients according to the International Germ Cell Cancer Collaborative Group (IGCCCG) risk classification.

7. Staging

Once a patient is diagnosed with a TGCTs the patient is staged with a through history and clinical examination. In the patients history it is important to ask the following questions with regards to the testicular lump. The crucial points in the history include the duration of symptoms, whether the lump is painful or painless, change in size of the lump, previous surgical history of UDT, sexual history , history of lower urinary tract symptoms and family history. Clinical examination includes assessment of supraclavicular lymph node, chest examination and abdominal examination for inguinal lymph nodes. At this stage a full set of Testicular tumour markers is performed which includes serum AFP, β-hCG and LDH is mandatory, while that of PLAP is optional. In cases of disseminated disease and life-threatening metastases, it is current practice to start with up-front chemotherapy, and orchidectomy may be delayed until clinical stabilisation has occurred.

In patients with a suspected testicular mass a radical inguinal orchidectomy is performed. The main principal of this procedure lies with exteriorisation of the testicle within its tunics. Prior to mobilization of the testis and cord, the cord is isolated and clamped to allow control of the draining lymphatics in order to minimize spillage and metastatic spread. If the diagnosis is not clear, a testicular biopsy (an enucleation of the intraparenchymal tumour) is taken for frozen section histological examination.

When the testicle is sent for pathological analysis, the EAU 2011 guidelines recommend a mandatory assessment of the specimen for the following features as these features further help prognosticate the patients outcome. The features include :-

1. Macroscopic features: side, testis size, maximum tumour size, and macroscopic features of epididymis, spermatic cord, and tunica vaginalis.
2. Sampling: a 1 cm^2 section for every centimetre of maximum tumour diameter, including normal macroscopic parenchyma (if present), albuginea and epididymis, with selection of suspected areas. At least one proximal and one distal section of spermatic cord plus any suspected area.
3. Microscopic features and diagnosis: histological type (specify individual components and estimate amount as percentage) according to WHO 2004 (11):-

a. Presence or absence of peri-tumoural venous and/or lymphatic invasion;
b. Presence or absence of albuginea, tunica vaginalis, rete testis, epididymis or spermatic cord invasion;
c. Presence or absence of intratubular germ cell neoplasia (IGCNU) in non-tumour parenchyma intratubular germ cell neoplasia.
d. pT category according to Tumour Node Metastasis (TNM) 2009.
e. Immunohistochemical studies: in seminoma and mixed germ cell tumour, AFP and hCG.

Following radical inguinal orchidectomy, the main aim of clinical staging is to determine whether the patient has metastatic or occult disease at the time of presentation. The investigations of choice to determine the above and accurately stage the TGCTs at presentation include the post-orchidectomy half-life kinetics of serum tumour markers; the status of retroperitoneal and supraclavicular lymph nodes, and the liver; the presence or absence of mediastinal nodal involvement and lung metastases; the status of brain and bone, if any suspicious symptoms are present. At this point all patients must have a serial testicular tumour markers measured and a thorough assessment of the retroperitoneum staging CT of the Chest, Abdomen and Pelvis. Retroperitoneal and mediastinal lymph nodes are best assessed by means of a CT scan. The supraclavicular nodes are best assessed by physical examination.

Hence, in Europe and the UK all patients with newly diagnosed TGCTs have the following invesigations performed:-

a. Serum testicular tumour markers (AFP, β-hCG and LDH)
b. CT - Chest, Abdomen and Pelvis
c. Ultrasound Testis (Bilateral)

A bone scan is organized in patients with suspected advances metastatic disease. A Brain CT is organized in patients In case of symptoms and patients with metastatic disease with multiple lung metastases and high beta-hCG levels. In some centre a detailed hormonal profile (Serum Testosterone, FSH, LH) and semen analysis is performed.

In all patients undergoing a radical inguinal orchidectomy it is important to counsel patients on the options of sperm banking and insertion of a testicular prosthesis. The 2011 EAU guidelines recommend cryopreservation of sperm prior to orchidectomy. This should be specifically offered in all patients with a history of Subfertility and atropic contralateral testis. In patients keen to pursue the insertion of a testicular prosthesis at the time of an inguinal orchidectomy, the risk of a possible delay to chemotherapy secondary to prosthesis related infection (0.6-2%) (24) must be highlighted.

7.1 Staging and prognostic classifications

The staging system recommended in these guidelines is the 2009 TNM of the International Union Against Cancer (UICC) (25) include the following parameters :-

a. Determination of the anatomical extent of disease
b. Assessment of serum tumour markers, including nadir values of hCG, AFP and LDH after orchidectomy (S category)
c. Clear definition of regional nodes
d. N-category modifications related to node size

The 2009 TNM of the International Union Against Cancer (UICC) is summarized in Table 1.

1. pT Primary tumour

pTX Primary tumour cannot be assessed

pT0 No evidence of primary tumour (e.g. histological scar in testis)

pTis Intratubular germ cell neoplasia (testicular intraepithelial neoplasia)

pT1 Tumour limited to testis and epididymis without vascular/lymphatic invasion: tumour may invade tunica albuginea but not tunica vaginalis

pT2 Tumour limited to testis and epididymis with vascular/lymphatic invasion, or tumour extending through tunica albuginea with involvement of tunica vaginalis

pT3 Tumour invades spermatic cord with or without vascular/lymphatic invasion pT4 Tumour invades scrotum with or without vascular/lymphatic invasion

2. Regional lymph nodes clinical

NX Regional lymph nodes cannot be assessed

N0 No regional lymph node metastasis

N1 Metastasis with a lymph node mass 2 cm or less in greatest dimension or multiple lymph nodes, none more than 2 cm in greatest dimension

N2 Metastasis with a lymph node mass more than 2 cm but not more than 5 cm in greatest dimension, or multiple lymph nodes, any one mass more than 2 cm but not more than 5 cm in greatest dimension

N3 Metastasis with a lymph node mass more than 5 cm in greatest dimension

3. pN Pathological

pNX Regional lymph nodes cannot be assessed

pN0 No regional lymph node metastasis

pN1 Metastasis with a lymph node mass 2 cm or less in greatest dimension and 5 or fewer positive nodes, none more than 2 cm in greatest dimension

pN2 Metastasis with a lymph node mass more than 2 cm but not more than 5 cm in greatest dimension; or more than 5 nodes positive, none more than 5 cm; or evidence or extranodal extension of tumour

pN3 Metastasis with a lymph node mass more than 5 cm in greatest dimension

4. M Distant metastasis

MX Distant metastasis cannot be assessed

M0 No distant metastasis

M1 Distant metastasis

M1a Non-regional lymph node(s) or lung

M1b Other sites

5. S Serum tumour markers

Sx Serum marker studies not available or not performed

S0 Serum marker study levels within normal limits

	LDH (U/l)	**hCG (mIU/ml)**	**AFP (ng/ml**
S1	<1.5 X N and	< 5000 and	< 1000
S2	1.5 - 10 X N or	5000 - 50,000 or	1,000-10,000
S3	> 10 X N or	> 50,000 or	> 10,000

Table 1.

On the attaining the TNMS information using the 2009 TNM of the International Union Against Cancer (UICC), patients are then staged using the American Joint Committee of Cancer (AJCC) staging classification (26) summarized in Table 2.

Stage 0	Stage I	Stage II	Stage III
pTis, N0, M0, S0	pT1-4, N0, M0, SX	Any pT/Tx, N1-3, M0, SX	Any pT/Tx, Any N, M1, SX
	Stage IA	**Stage IIA**	**Stage IIIA**
	pT1, N0, M0, S0	Any pT/Tx, N1, M0, S0	Any pT/Tx, Any N, M1a, S0
		Any pT/Tx, N1, M0, S1	Any pT/Tx, Any N, M1a, S1
	Stage IB	**Stage IIB**	**Stage IIIB**
	pT2, N0, M0, S0	Any pT/Tx, N2, M0, S0	Any pT/Tx, N1-3, M0, S2
	pT3, N0, M0, S0	Any pT/Tx, N2, M0, S1	Any pT/Tx, Any N, M1a, S2
	pT4, N0, M0, S0		
	Stage IC	**Stage IIC**	**Stage IIIC**
	Any pT/Tx, N0, M0, S1-3	Any pT/Tx, N3, M0, S0	Any pT/Tx, N1-3, M0, S3
		Any pT/Tx, N3, M0, S1	Any pT/Tx, Any N, M1a, S3
			Any pT/Tx, Any N, M1b, Any S

Table 2. The AJCC staging groupings of Testicular Tumours

8. Management

Within Europe and the UK the management of TGCTs differs mainly for the indications of Retroperitoneal Lymph Node Dissection (RPLND) in both Stage I and Stage II disease. We classify the management of TGCTs as followed in Europe and the UK based on whether the tumour is a Seminoma or Non-Seminoma.

8.1 Management of Seminoma

Of all Seminomas diagnosed, 75% are confined to the testicle itself at the time of clinical presentation and a complete cure is thus achieved with a thorough radical inguinal orchidectomy. In upto 10-15% of patients metastasis is present at the time of diagnosis with a further 5-10% of patients having more advanced disease.

In patients with Non-metastatic Stage I seminoma (T1N0M0S0-1) the risk of subsequent para-aortic lymph node relapse is 20%. Adjuvant therapy with either chemotherapy or radiotherapy reduces the risk of recurrence to <1%.

8.1.1 Management of stage I Seminoma

The options in a patient with Stage 1 Seminoma include surveillance, adjuvant chemotherapy or adjuvant radiotherapy. The option of surveillance is indicated as 75% of Seminoma are cured following a radical inguinal orchidectomy. In a large study of 1500 patients (28) indicated the overall rate of retroperitoneal disease relapse to be 16.8%. It is important to characterize patients with high risk Stage I Seminoma based on initial pathology. The 2 most important factors associated with poor prognosis includes the presence of rete-testis invasion and tumours size of ≥ 4 cm. The overall cancer-specific survival rate reported with surveillance performed by experienced centres is 97-100% for seminoma stage I (29-31). The main drawback of surveillance is the need for more intensive follow-up, especially with repeated imaging examinations of the retroperitoneal lymph nodes, for at least 5 years after orchidectomy.

Prognostic Group	Progression free survival (PFS) and overall survival (OS)	Clinical Criteria
Good prognostic group (Non Seminoma)	*Non-seminoma (56% of cases)* 5-year PFS 89% 5-year survival 92%	*All of the following criteria:* • Testis/retroperitoneal primary • No non-pulmonary visceral metastases • AFP < 1,000 ng/mL • hCG < 5,000 IU/L (1,000 ng/mL) • LDH < 1.5 x ULN
Good prognostic group (Seminoma)	*Seminoma (90% of cases)* 5-year PFS 82% 5-year survival 86%	*All of the following criteria:* • Testis/retroperitoneal primary • No non-pulmonary visceral metastases • AFP < 1,000 ng/mL • hCG < 5,000 IU/L (1,000 ng/mL) • LDH < 1.5 x ULN
Intermediate prognosis group (Non Seminoma)	*Non-seminoma (28% of cases)* 5 years PFS 75% 5-year survival 80%	• Testis/retroperitoneal primary • No non-pulmonary visceral metastases • AFP 1,000 - 10,000 ng/mL or • hCG 5,000 - 50,000 IU/L or • LDH 1.5 - 10 x ULN
Intermediate prognosis group (Seminoma)	*Seminoma (10% of cases)* 5-year PFS 67% 5-year survival 72%	*Any of the following criteria:* • Any primary site • Non-pulmonary visceral metastases • Normal AFP • Any hCG • Any LDH
Poor prognosis group (Non Seminoma)	*Non-seminoma (16% of cases)* 5-year PFS 41% 5-year survival 48%	*Any of the following criteria:* • Mediastinal primary • Non-pulmonary visceral metastases • AFP > 10,000 ng/mL or • hCG > 50,000 IU/L (10,000 ng/mL) or • LDH > 10 x ULN
Poor prognosis group (Seminoma)	No patients classified as poor prognosis	N/A

Table 3. Prognostic-based staging system for metastatic germ cell cancer (International Germ Cell Cancer Collaborative Group).

Patients with Stage I Seminoma can also be given adjuvant chemotherapy with one cycle of Carboplatin (33). An alternative to surveillance or chemotherapy in patients with radiotherapy (34).

Within Europe and the UK, a RPLND is not recommended in patients with Stage 1 Seminoma. In prospective, non-randomised study comparing radiotherapy and RPLND in stage I seminoma, there was a trend towards a higher incidence of retroperitoneal relapses (9.5%) after RPLND as primary treatment (35).

In summary, it is important to stratify patients with Stage 1 Seminoma into high risk based on the presence of rete testis invasion and tumour volume of ≥ 4 cm. In these patients the option of adjuvant chemotherapy and radiotherapy is justifiable. In patients without rete testis invasion or in whom the testicular tumour volume is ≤ 4 cm the option of surveillance alone is recommended.

8.1.2 Management of stage II Seminoma

The options in a patient with Stage II Seminoma is radiotherapy. However, chemotherapy is an alternative management strategy.

8.2 Management of Non-Seminoma

In patients with Non-Seminomas, 30% with Stage I disease will have subclinical metastases and will relapse if surveillance alone is applied following orchidectomy. Within this groups of patients the options of treatment include surveillance, chemotherapy and RPLND. It is important to stratify Non-Seminomas into high risk based tumours depeding on the following parameters which include the presence of Vascular/lymphatic in or peri-tumoural invasion, proliferation rate > 70% or percentage of embryonal carcinoma > 50%.

8.2.1 Management of stage I Non-Seminoma

In patients on surveillance, the incidence of relapse is 30% (36). When a patient relapses about 35% have normal levels of serum tumour markers at relapse and approximately 60% of relapses are within the retroperitoneum. Upto 11% of relapsing patients have large-volume recurrent disease at representation. Based on the above, the option of surveillance should be offered to a compliant patient who will agree for very regular and close follow up.

The commonest option of management of patients within Europe and the UK with Stage I Non-Seminoma is chemotherapy. The current recommendation is two courses of chemotherapy with cisplatin, etoposide and bleomycin (PEB) as primary treatment for high-risk patients (having about 50% risk of relapse). Patient receiving adjuvant chemotherapy must be monitored closely as there is a risk of slow-growing retroperitoneal teratomas after primary chemotherapy.

A Nerve sparing / template based RPLND can also be offered to patient who are not keen to receive chemotherapy. It is interesting to note that about 30% of patients are diagnosed to have a retroperitoneal lymph node metastases corresponding to pathological stage II (PS2) disease. In patients with no retroperitoneal metastases found at RPLND (PS1), approximately 10% of the PS1 patients relapse at distant sites. Within the UK, RPLND is normally indicated in post chemotherapy recurrence.

As with seminomas a further risk adaptive strategy can be adapted for Non-Seminomas. If the risk-adapted policy is applied, patients with vascular invasion are recommended to undergo adjuvant chemotherapy with two cycles of PEB, and patients without vascular invasion are recommended to undergo surveillance. In summary patients with CS1A (pT1, no vascular invasion), low risk Stage I Non Seminoma can be offered the option of surveillance. If patients are not willing (or suitable) to undergo surveillance, adjuvant chemotherapy or nerve-sparing RPLND are alternative treatment options. If RPLND reveals PN+ (nodal involvement) disease, chemotherapy with two courses of PEB should be considered. Patients with Stage I Non-Seminoma CS1B (pT2-pT4) high risk disease receive either primary chemotherapy with two courses of PEB or Surveillance or nerve-sparing RPLND in high-risk patients remain options for those not willing to undergo adjuvant chemotherapy.

8.2.2 Management of stage II Non-Seminoma

In patients with Stage II Non-Seminoma with normal testicular tumour markers can be managed with primary RPLND or surveillance. In patients with elevated tumour markers primary chemotherapy is recommended. When surveillance is commenced for a lesion the lesion can either regress, resolve or progress with either a rise or no rise in concomitant testicular markers.

When a lesion regresses in the absence of rising tumour markers it is unlikely to be a malignancy. A lesion growing represents either a teratoma or a well differentiated tumour in the absence of rising testicular tumour markers. In this situation a RPLND should be performed by an experienced surgeon. Patients with a growing lesion and a concomitant increase in tumour markers AFP or beta-hCG should not undergo surgery. These patients require chemotherapy with PEB according to the treatment algorithm for patients with metastatic disease and IGCCCG. Patients who are unwilling to commence primary chemotherapy have an option of a nerve-sparing RPLND with adjuvant chemotherapy (two cycles of PEB) in case of metastatic disease (pII A/B).

9. Follow up

Follow-up care with an oncologist, urologist or both, is vital for the patient with testicular cancer. Regular assessments are required to monitor tumour markers in the blood, chest X-rays, CT scans of the abdomen and a full medical examination with psychological support. This process may continue for several years and may vary depending on the type and stage of the disease.

10. Conclusion

In conclusion the management of TGCTs within the UK and Europe is based on the individuals management (surveillance, chemotherapy or radiotherapy) which has to be balanced according to clinical features and the risk of short-term and long-term toxic effects. Although cure rates for Stage 1 disease are high, there continues to be significant morbidity due to chemotherapy, RPLND and Radiotherapy for concomitant additional treatment. We recommend individualizing patient treatment using a Multidisciplinary team approach using the latest regional, national and international guidelines and developments.

11. Abbreviations

TGCTs	Testicular Germ Cell tumours
PGC	Primordial germ cells
UDT	Undescended Testis
IGCNU	Intratubular germ cell neoplasia
MOE	Maternal Oestrogen Exposure

HCG Human chorionic gonadotrophin

AFP Alpha-fetoprotein

LDH Lactate dehydrogenase

PLAP Placental alkaline phosphatase

IGCCCG International Germ Cell Cancer Collaborative Group

AJCC American Joint Committee of Cancer

RPLND Retroperitoneal Lymph Node Dissection

12. References

Aparicio J, García del Muro X, Maroto P, et al.Spanish Germ Cell Cancer Cooperative Group (GG). Multicenter study evaluating a dual policy of postorchidectomy surveillance and selective adjuvant single-agent carboplatin for patients with clinical stage I seminoma. Ann Oncol 2003 Jun;14(6):867-72.

Bode PK, Barghorn A, Fritzsche FR, Riener MO, Kristiansen G, Knuth A, Moch H. MAGEC2 is a sensitive and novel marker for seminoma: a tissue microarray analysis of 325 testicular germ cell tumours. Mod Pathol. 2011 Jun;24(6):829-35

Bosl GJ, Motzer RJ. Testicular germ-cell cancer. N Engl J Med 1997 Nov;337(4):242-53.

Calvert AH, Newell DR, Gumbrell LA, et al. Carboplatin dosage: prospective evaluation of a simple formula based on renal function. J Clin Oncol. 1989;7:1748-1756.

Cancer Incidence in Five Continents, Vol IX. Curado MP, Edwards B, Shin R, et al eds. IARC Scientific Publication 2007, No. 160.

Cassidy FH, Ishioka KM, McMahon CJ, et al. MR imaging of scrotal tumors and pseudotumors. Radiographics 2010 May; 30(3):665-83.

Chung P, Parker C, Panzarella T, et al. Surveillance in stage I testicular seminoma-risk of late relapse. Can J Urol 2002 Oct;9(5):1637-40.

Engholm G, Ferlay J, Christensen N, et al. NORDCAN--a Nordic tool for cancer information, planning, quality control and research. Acta Oncol 2010 Jun;49(5):725-36

Fosså SD, Horwich A, Russell JM, et al. Optimal planning target volume for stage I testicular seminoma: A Medical Research Council Testicular Tumor Working Group randomized trial. J Clin Oncol 1999 Apr;17(4):1146

Freedman LS, Parkinson MC, Jones WG, et al. Histopathology in the prediction of relapse of patients with stage I testicular teratoma treated by orchidectomy alone. Lancet 1987 Aug;2(8554):294-8.

Henderson BE, Benton B, Jing J, Yu MC, Pike MC. Risk factors for cancer of the testis in young men. Int J Cancer. 1979 May 15;23(5):598-602.

Horwich, A., Shipley, J. & Huddart, R. Testicular germ-cell cancer. Lancet 367, 754–765 (2006)

Huyghe E, Matsuda T, Thonneau P. Increasing incidence of testicular cancer worldwide: a review. J Urol 2003 Jul;170(1):5-11.

International Germ Cell Cancer Collaborative Group. International Germ Cell Consensus Classification: a prognostic factor-based staging system for metastatic germ cell cancers. J Clin Oncol 1997 Feb;15(2):594-603.

Kanetsky PA, Mitra N, Vardhanabhuti S, et al. Common variation in KITLG and at 5q31.3 predisposes to testicular germ cell cancer. Nat Genet 2009 Jul;41(7):811-5.

Kim W, Rosen MA, Langer JE, et al. US-MR Imaging correlation in pathologic conditions of the scrotum. Radiographics 2007 Sep-Oct; 27(5):1239-53.

Korkola JE, Houldsworth J, Feldman DR, et al. Identification and validation of a gene expression signature that predicts outcome in adult men with germ cell tumors. J Clin Oncol 2009 Nov 1;27(31):5240-7.

La Vecchia C, Bosetti C, Lucchini F, et al. Cancer Mortality in Europe, 2000-2004, and an overview of trends since 1995. Ann Oncol. 2010 Jun; 21(6):1323-60. Epub 2009 Nov 30

Looijenga LH, Gillis AJ, Stoop H, et al. Relevance of microRNAs in normal and malignant development, including human testicular germ cell tumours. Int J Androl 2007 Aug;30(4):304-14; discussion 314-15.

Marshall S. Potential problems with testicular prostheses. Urology. 1986 Nov;28(5):388-90

Oliver RT, Mason MD, Mead GM, et al. MRC TE19 collaborators and the EORTC 30982 collaborators. Radiotherapy versus single-dose carboplatin in adjuvant treatment of stage I seminoma: a randomised trial. Lancet 2005 Jul;23-29;366(9482):293-300.

Oosterhuis, J. W. & Looijenga, L. H. Testicular germ-cell tumours in a broader perspective. Nature Rev. Cancer 5, 210–222 (2005).

Peyret C. Tumeurs du testicule. Synthèse et recommendations en onco-urologie. Prog Urol 1993;2:60-4.

Rapley EA, Turnbull C, Al Olama AA, et al; UK Testicular Cancer Collaboration. A genome-wide association study of testicular germ cell tumor. Nat Genet 2009 Jul;41(7):807-10.

Reuter VE. Origins and molecular biology of testicular germ cell tumors. Mod Pathol 2005 Feb;18(Suppl 2):S51-S60.

Schottenfeld D, Warshauer ME, Sherlock S, Zauber AG, Leder M, Payne R. The epidemiology of testicular cancer in young adults. Am J Epidemiol. 1980 Aug;112(2):232-46

Skakkebaek NE, Berthelsen JG, Müller J. Carcinoma-in-situ of the undescended testis. Urol Clin North Am. 1982 Oct;9(3):377-85

Sobin LH, Gospodariwicz M, Wittekind C (eds). TNM classification of malignant tumors. UICC International Union Against Cancer, 7th edn. Wiley-Blackwell, 2009 Dec; pp 249-254.

Tandstad T, Smaaland R, Solberg A, et al. Management of Seminomatous Testicular Cancer: A Binational Prospective Population-Based Study From the Swedish Norwegian Testicular Cancer Study Group (SWENOTECA). J Clin Oncol. 2011 Jan 4

Testis. In: American Joint Committee on Cancer: AJCC Cancer Staging Manual. Philadelphia, Pa: Lippincott-Raven Publishers, 5th ed., 1997, pp 225-230.

Thornhill JA, Conroy RM, Kelly DG, Walsh A, Fennelly JJ, Fitzpatrick JM. Public awareness of testicular cancer and the value of self examination. Br Med J 1986;293(6545):480-1.

Thornhill JA, Fennelly JJ , Kelly DG, Walsh A, Fitzpatrick JM.Patients' delay in the presentation of testis cancer in Ireland. Br J Urol 1987;59(5):447-51.

Wanderas EH, Tretli S, Fossa SD. Trends in incidence of testicular cancer in Norway 1955-1992. Eur J Cancer 1995 Nov;31A(12):2044-8.

Warde P, Jewett MAS. Surveillance for stage I testicular seminoma. Is it a good option? Urol Clin North Am 1998 Aug;25(3):425-33.

Warszawski N, Schmucking M. Relapses in early-stage testicular seminoma: radiation therapy versus retroperitoneal lymphadenectomy. Scan J Urol Nephrol 1997 Aug;31(4):335-9.

WHO histological classification of testis tumours, In: Eble JN, Sauter G, Epstein JI, Sesterhenn IA, eds.Pathology & Genetics. Tumours of the urinary system and male genital organs. Lyons: IARC Press, 2004: 218, pp. 250-262.

Part 2

Scientific Perspectives

5

Mouse Models of Testicular Germ Cell Tumors

Delphine Carouge and Joseph H. Nadeau
Institute for Systems Biology
Seattle, Washington
USA

1. Introduction

Germ cell tumors arise from anomalies in primordial germ cells (PGCs) (Stevens, 1967), the embryonic precursors of oocytes and sperm. Their normal development follows three steps: migration, proliferation and differentiation into mature germ cells (Mauduit et al., 1999). Abnormalities in these steps can result in sterility, reduced fertility, or in some cases to transformation into ovarian tumors in females or testicular germ cell tumors (TGCTs) in males (Stevens, 1967), both of which present remarkable cellular and tissue heterogeneity reflecting the pluripotent nature of the TGCT stem cell.

Although representing only 1-2% of all cancers in men, TGCTs are the most common malignancy affecting young men 15-35 years of age (Buetow, 1995). Over the past decade, TGCT incidence has risen ~1.2% per year with about 8,300-8,400 new cases reported in the United States (American Cancer Society, www.cancer.org). TGCT risk varies more than 5-fold among ethnic groups and geographic regions (McGlynn et al., 2005; www.cancer.org). In addition, developmental anomalies such as undescended testis are indicators of TGCT risk (Dieckmann & Pichlmeier, 2004). Finally, environmental factors such as pesticides or insecticides strongly influence susceptibility. However, the mechanisms by which genetic and environmental factors affect susceptibility remain elusive.

Genetic factors account for 25% of susceptibility to TGCTs, making these tumors the third most heritable cancer (Gilbert et al., 2011). Family history is a significant risk factor with 8- to 10-fold risk for brothers of men with TGCTs and 4- to 6-fold risk for sons (Hutter et al., 1967). The risk increases 75-fold for monozygotic twins (Swerdlow et al., 1999). Genome-wide association studies (GWAS) in humans reveal various loci that contribute to susceptibility, but the identity of these genes has not yet been established (Gilbert et al., 2011). Discovery of TGCTs in the 129 family of inbred strains of mice has enabled identification and characterization of specific genes and their interactions (Stevens & Little, 1954; Stevens, 1973).

In this chapter, after discussing the various mouse models for TGCTs, we review the evidence for TGCT genes and their role in tumorigenesis in both humans and mice. We consider the consequence of their mutation, as well as the role of gene interactions, to better understand molecular pathways of PGC transformation and pathogenesis. Finally, we discuss evidence for transgenerational effects that influence TGCT incidence.

2. Mouse models for human TGCTs

Studies of TGCT development before birth are not feasible in humans. Laboratory mice therefore provide unique opportunities to determine the genetic basis for TGCT susceptibility and for characterizing key components contributing to PGC transformation.

2.1 TGCT predisposition in the 129 inbred strain

During gastrulation in the mouse embryo, PGCs arise from the ectoderm and the precursors of Leydig and Sertoli cells arise from the coelomic epithelium (Clark & Eddy, 1975; Karl & Capel, 1998). At 8 days post-coitum (E8), 50-100 PGCs are evident at the base of the allantois where they begin to be highly mobile (Fig. 1) (Clark & Eddy, 1975; Molyneaux et al., 2001). From E9.5 onwards, PGCs rapidly exit the hind-gut epithelium and migrate toward the genital ridges (Molyneaux et al., 2001). During migration, PGCs proliferate reaching a maximum of 20,000-25,000 cells at E13.5 (Mauduit et al., 1999). Then, in males, PGCs become quiescent (mitotic arrest) and are called gonocytes (Mauduit et al., 1999). Pre-Sertoli cells appear in male gonads around E11 for playing roles in: (1) sex determination because of their SRY factor released (Albrecht & Eicher, 2001); (2) migration of PGCs depending on chemotactic factors (i.e. KITLG, a specific-Sertoli factor) and germ-Sertoli interactions (Griswold, 1995); and (3) the arrest of male germ cell mitosis in G1/S phase (Karl & Capel, 1998). Mitotic arrest is maintained until three days after the birth (P3) (Mauduit et al., 1999).

At P6, gonocytes differentiate into Type A1 spermatogonia and begin radial migration in the seminiferous tubule (Nagano et al., 2000). Germ cells undergo either a proliferative period (to maintain the progenitor population throughout the reproductive life of males) or meiosis (to mature germ cells) (Nagano et al., 2000). During these postnatal days, pre-Sertoli cells transform into mature Sertoli cells that support germ cell differentiation and spermatogenesis (Griswold, 1995; Hess et al., 2006). Remarkably, a significant proportion of PGCs remains scattered along the migratory route. These ectopic PGCs are eliminated between E10 and E17 by activating the intrinsic cell death pathway (Stallock et al., 2003). This intrinsic pathway is regulated by BCL2 family members (i.e. BAX, BAK and BCL2), which activate mitochondria leading to secretion of cytochrome C, an initiator of apoptosis (Shimizu et al., 1999; Stallock et al., 2003). Another BAX-dependent apoptotic control point occurs at P10-P13 before meiosis to eliminate germ cells that fail either to migrate in the seminiferous tubules or to repair DNA (de Rooij, 2001).

In the 129 family of inbred strains, 5%-10% of males develop spontaneous TGCTs (Fig. 1) (Stevens & Little, 1954; Stevens, 1967), making these strains highly relevant for learning about TGCT development in humans. Indeed, TGCTs in mice are most similar to pediatric TGCTs in humans, and both species have a similar left-sided preference of the tumors. Bilateral TGCTs are infrequent in mice and usually involve less than 5% of all cases in humans (Dieckmann & Pichlmeier, 2004). The critical period for transformation is between E11.5-E13.5 in mice (Stevens & Little, 1954; Stevens, 1967). Interestingly, syncytial masses of atypical gonocytes are detected in embryonic testis cords from E13 onward in 129 wild-type and mutant males (Stevens, 1967; T. Noguchi & M. Noguchi, 1985; Rivers & Hamilton, 1986; Matin et al., 1999). These atypical cells may result from incomplete cell cycle, mitotic arrest defects, or de-differentiation after their entrance in quiescence (Rivers & Hamilton, 1986).

These so-called embryonal carcinoma (EC) cells escape necrosis, and then proliferate and aggregate together to form clusters, which are correlated with partial or complete germ cell deficiency (Stevens, 1967; T. Noguchi & M. Noguchi, 1985; Rivers & Hamilton, 1986; Matin et al., 1999). Furthermore, EC clusters have been suggested as the precursors of either testicular abnormalities, which have been found in an appreciable frequency (18%) in 129 males, or TGCTs (Rivers & Hamilton, 1986). Similar abnormalities, termed carcinoma in situ, have been found in humans many years before invasive malignancy (Skakkebaek, 1972). Why some germ cells transform into EC clusters while others develop normally is unclear, just as why some abnormal gonocytes die while others persist.

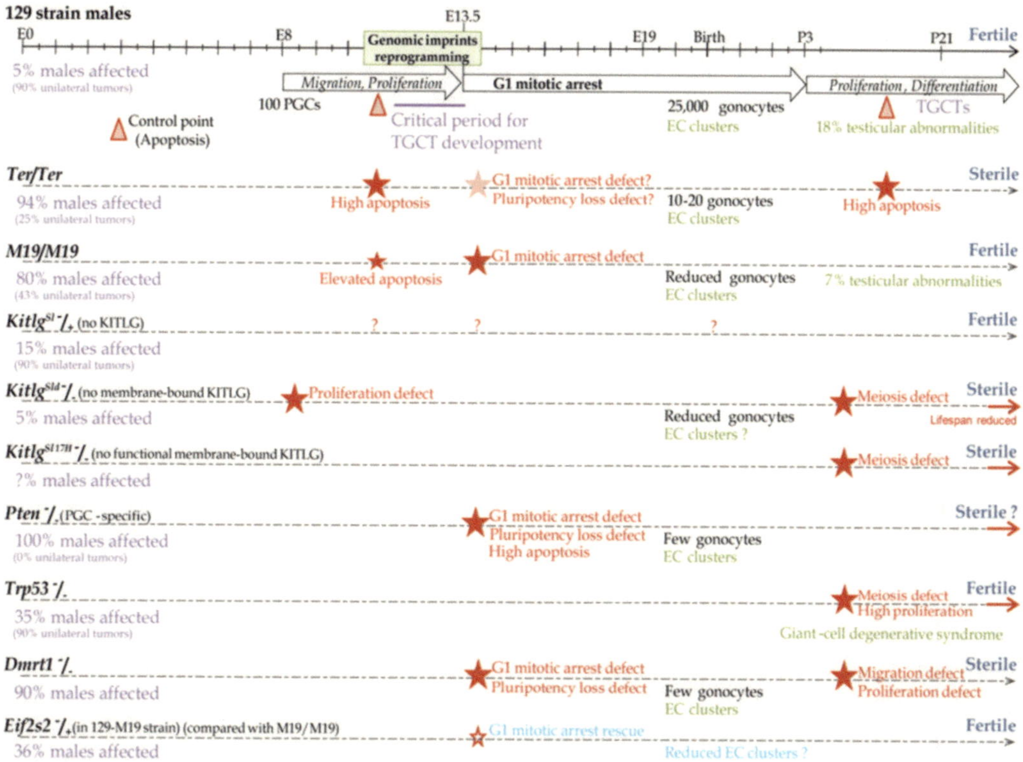

Fig. 1. Male germ cell development in mouse models for TGCTs in the 129 strain.

2.2 TGCTs in the 129-*Ter* strain

The *Ter* allele, also known as *Teratoma,* has dramatic effects on PGC biology and TGCT susceptibility (Stevens, 1973; T. Noguchi & M. Noguchi, 1985), and was recently identified as a spontaneous mutation in the *Dead-end* (*Dnd1*) gene (Youngren et al., 2005). *Ter* homozygosity causes severe germ cell deficiency in both sexes, probably mediated through BAX-dependent apoptosis after E8.5 (Stevens, 1973; T. Noguchi & M. Noguchi, 1985; Cook et al., 2009). EC clusters develop from E13 in 129-*Ter*/*Ter* male embryos probably due to a defect in G1/S mitotic arrest (Rivers & Hamilton, 1986). The few surviving PGCs successfully migrate to the genital ridges, suggesting that DND1 is not essential for migration (Youngren et al., 2005). Deficiency progresses with age until P11 when PGCs are no longer detectable (T. Noguchi & M. Noguchi, 1985; Cook et al., 2009). As a result, adult mutant males are sterile (Fig. 1) (T. Noguchi & M. Noguchi, 1985). Somatic development of Sertoli and Leydig progenitors is not affected in accordance with the PGC-specific expression of *Dnd1* (Weidinger et al., 2003). Interestingly, 17% of 129-*Ter*/+ males develop tumors, 10% of which are bilateral, but these males are fertile. This rate increases to 94% in homozygotes with 75% of cases having bilateral tumors (T. Noguchi & M. Noguchi, 1985).

DND1 was originally proposed to be a component of the cytidine to uridine RNA editing complex given its similarity with the Apobec complementation factor (A1CF) (Weidinger et al., 2003). More recently, DND1 was shown to block miRNA access to their mRNA targets (Kedde et al., 2007). The reactivated target genes are involved in PGC pluripotency (i.e. *Sox2*, *Nanos1* and *Nanog*), in cell cycle regulation (i.e. *Cyclin-dependent kinase inhibitors (Cdkn) 1b*, *Cdkn1a*) and in PGC survival (i.e. *Transformation related protein* (*Trp53*), apoptotic factor *Bax* and *Phosphatase and tensin homolog* (*Pten*)) (Kedde et al., 2007; Cook et al., 2011; R. Zhu et al., 2011). *Dnd1* is expressed throughout embryogenesis with an up-regulation between E12.5 and E15.5 in males, the critical period for TGCT development (Youngren et al., 2005; Cook et al., 2009). Thus, loss of DND1 in *Ter* mutants strongly affects differentiation, survival and entry in quiescence of PGCs and dramatically enhances the TGCT frequency in the 129 strain.

2.3 Consomic 129 inbred strains

Chromosome Substitution Strains (CSSs, consomic strains) carry entire chromosomes derived from another inbred strain. Some CSSs were created to study the genetic linkage of the MOLF-derived TGCT modifier genes. MOLF is derived from *Mus musculus molossinus,* which is genetically distinct from 129 and has no predisposition for TGCTs (Mieno et al., 1989; Matin et al., 1998). We will review results for two consomic strains.

2.3.1 129-M18

The 129-M18 CSS substitutes MOLF-derived chromosome 18 for its homologue in 129 wild-type mice (Anderson et al., 2009a). 129-M18 males show complete resistance to develop TGCTs with no homozygous males affected. Four quantitative trait loci (QTLs, Region I-IV) were identified independent of the *Dnd1* gene, which is also located on this chromosome.

Region I shows homology with the 10p11 region in humans (Copeland et al., 1993). One candidate gene may be *Map3k8,* which encodes a mitogen-activated protein kinase (MAPK) that acts downstream of tyrosine kinase-dependent pathway (Patriotis et al., 1994). Region II belongs to a conserved region 5q in humans (Copeland et al., 1993). In mice, this region contains *Eif1a* gene, which encodes a translational regulator that is functionally related to eIF2α, encoded by *Eif2s2* gene, loss of which suppresses TGCT development (Heaney et al., 2009) (Section 3.5). However, the three homologues of *Eif1a* gene are *EIF1AD* on chromosome 11, and *EIF1AX* and *EIF1AY* on sex chromosomes in humans. Region III contains at least one TGCT enhancer and is conserved with the 18q region in humans (Copeland et al., 1993). An interesting candidate gene is *Noxa,* which encodes a mitochondria-mediated apoptotic factor (Krishna et al., 2011). Interestingly, *Noxa* is activated by the TGCT suppressor TRP53 (Michalak et al., 2005; Donehower et al., 1992)

(Section 3.3). Region IV contains the *F-box only protein 15* gene, one of the few known targets of the stem cell pluripotent factor OCT3/4 (Tokuzawa et al., 2003).

2.3.2 129-M19

The 129-M19 CSS substitutes MOLF-derived chromosome 19 for its homolog in 129 wild-type mice (Matin et al., 1999). Surprisingly, 80% of the homosomic males develop TGCTs and this unusually high tumor frequency remain elevated (20%) when only one copy of M19 is present (129-M19/+) compared with 129 wild-type mice (5%), suggesting a semi-dominant effect of the MOLF susceptibility locus (Matin et al., 1999; Youngren et al., 2003). In contrast with the 129-*Ter* strain, M19 does not cause complete germ cell deficiency (Fig. 1). Indeed, some PGCs can develop normally leading to fertility in both homozygous and heterozygous males. Furthermore, the incidence of bilateral tumors in 129-M19/M19 is reduced (57%) compared with the 129-*Ter* strain (75%) and are non-existent in heterozygous males (similar than in 129 wild type males) (Matin et al., 1999; Youngren et al., 2003). Thus, the phenotype of this consomic M19 strain is less severe than in the 129-*Ter* strain.

Regions on chromosome 19 are homologous to either 9p, which contains the TGCT modifier *doublesex- & Mab3-related transcription factor 1* (*Dmrt1*) gene (Section 3.4), 9q, 10q, which contains the TGCT modifier *Pten* (Section 3.2) and 11q in humans (Copeland et al., 1993). An interesting candidate gene is *Splicing factor 1* (*Sf1*), which encodes an RNA binding protein that functions as a pre-mRNA splicing factor (Z. Liu et al., 2001). Interestingly, *Sf1* deficiency (heterozygous *Sf1*$^{-}$/$_{+}$) in 129-M19/+ males reduces the incidence of TGCTs (R. Zhu et al., 2010), suggesting that *Sf1* may be one of the TGCT enhancer genes on chromosome 19. *D19Bwg1357e* is a predicted gene down-regulated in the gonads of MOLF strain mice (R. Zhu et al., 2007). This gene has an RNA-binding domain homologous to those in *Pum1* and *Pum2* genes, which encode two major components of P-bodies, the center of RNA processing (Moore et al., 2003), suggesting a similar role for *D19Bwg1357e*.

Thus, CSSs are powerful tools for identifying new genes that, alone or in combination and with conventional additive or epistatic effects, confer susceptibility to TGCTs. These candidate genes are involved in RNA biology, epigenetic regulation and intracellular pathways regulating PGC survival, proliferation and pluripotency.

3. TGCT modifier genes in the 129 strain

Spontaneous and engineered mutations are essential for characterizing molecular pathways involved in PGC development and transformation into TGCTs. In this section, we review the phenotypic traits of 129 mice that carry mutations on TGCT modifier genes.

3.1 *Kit* and *Kitlg*

In the mouse, mutations at the *White-spotting* (W) or *Steel* (Sl) loci cause sterility and severe anemia that lead to *in utero* or perinatal death in homozygotes (McCoshen & McCallion, 1975; Nocka et al., 1990). The *W* locus, located on chromosome 5 in mice (region 4q12 in humans), encodes KIT, a tyrosine kinase receptor (Manova et al., 1990). The ligand of KIT, named KITLG, is encoded at the *Sl* locus on chromosome 10 in mice (region 12q21 in humans) (Flanagan et al., 1991). These two factors are essential for hematopoiesis, melanogenesis and gametogenesis (Bernstein et al., 1991; Besmer et al., 1993).

In the testis, KIT is expressed on the surface of PGCs from E7.5 to E13.5, and then at P5, on differentiating germ cells and interstitial Leydig cells (Manova et al., 1990; Yoshinaga et al., 1991). KITLG is only expressed by the pre-Sertoli and Sertoli cells (Rossi et al., 1991; Tajima et al., 1991). The two forms of KITLG, soluble and membrane-bound, are differentially expressed depending on developmental stages (Matsui et al., 1990; Flanagan et al., 1991; E.J. Huang et al., 1992). The membrane-bound KITLG is predominantly expressed during proliferative periods: between E8 and E14 and just after the birth (P3), and the soluble form when PGCs are quiescent (between E13.5 and P3) (Matsui et al., 1990; Flanagan et al., 1991; E.J. Huang et al., 1992). In addition of their essential role during migration, the interaction of KITLG with its receptor leads to the dimerization of KIT and its auto-phosphorylation activates two major pathways: (1) the PI3K/AKT signaling cascade regulates transcription of mitotic inhibitors such as CDKN1a, CDKN1b and cyclin D1, and enhances the translational factor eIF4E; (2) the MAPK pathway regulates factors involved in pluripotency such as NANOG and SOX2, and in proliferation (Mithraprabhu & Loveland, 2009). By acting on TRP53 activity, KIT/KITLG pathway controls apoptosis of PGCs by regulating the BCL2 components (i.e. BAX, BAK, BCL2) and their cofactors (i.e. PUMA, NOXA) (Pesce et al., 1993; Carson et al., 1994), explaining why ectopic PGCs that lose KIT/KITLG interaction in 129 wild-type mice are eliminated by apoptosis.

Loss of KIT (Kit^{W} and Kit^{Wv}) or KITLG ($Kitlg^{Sl}$, $Kitlg^{SlJ}$ and $Kitlg^{Slgb}$) leads to massive PGC loss, resulting from high levels of apoptosis beginning on or before E9 (Stevens, 1967; McCoshen & McCallion, 1975; Nocka et al., 1990; Heaney et al., 2008). In these *Kit* and *Kitlg* heterozygous mutants, the wild-type allele is sufficient to rescue PGC viability at E13.5 and fertility in adult males. Loss of only membrane-bound KITLG in the $Kitlg^{Sld}$ deletion leads to a mild phenotype characterized by partial PGC deficiency because of a proliferation defect (Fig. 1) (Flanagan et al., 1991; Tajima et al., 1991). At later stages, this mutation adversely affects PGC differentiation resulting in sterility. In $Kitlg^{Sl17H}$ mutants, the membrane-bound form is not functional due to absence of its cytoplasmic tail (Brannan et al., 1992). These mutants present a slight phenotype apparent after birth with anomalies in spermatogenesis, leading to sterility (Fig. 1). Surprisingly, $Kitlg^{Sld}$ and $Kitlg^{Sl17H}$ mutants have normal apoptosis when mice lacking KIT or KITLG have a high apoptotic rate, suggesting that soluble KITLG alone is sufficient to re-establishing normal apoptosis (Flanagan et al., 1991; Brannan et al., 1992). Nonetheless, neither $Kitlg^{Sld}$ nor $Kitlg^{Sl17H}$ mutants are fertile, suggesting that membrane-bound KITLG is necessary for complete PGC development (proliferation and differentiation). Thus, the KIT/KITLG pathway controls the migration, proliferation and survival of PGCs during embryogenesis, and the proliferation, differentiation and the radial development of germ cells after birth.

Although loss of KIT and KITLG have similar effects on PGC development, only $Kitlg^{Sl}$, $Kitlg^{SlJ}$ and $Kitlg^{Slgb}$ heterozygotes have 2-fold increase in occurrence of TGCT-affected males (Fig. 1) (Stevens, 1967; Heaney et al., 2008), suggesting that KIT is haplosufficient to promote TGCT formation. Interestingly, $Kitlg^{Sld}$ allele has no effect on TGCT susceptibility (Heaney et al., 2008), suggesting that soluble KITLG is sufficient to suppress TGCT formation. The presence of EC clusters and the frequency of testicular abnormalities in $Kitlg^{Sl}$ and Kit^{W}

heterozygous males remain to be evaluated. However, given that EC clusters are probably the origin of TGCTs and that some clusters have been described in mice lacking the PI3K binding site on KIT (Kissel et al., 2000), we expect to find EC clusters at least in *Kitlg*^{Sl}, *Kitlg*^{SlJ} and *Kitlg*^{Slgb} heterozygous males. Determining whether soluble KITLG in *Kitlg*^{Sld} mutants reduces the frequency of these clusters, or whether *Kit*^{W} mutants also carry EC clusters without transformation into tumors, could highlight the molecular pathway involved in transformation of benign EC masses into malignant tumors.

3.2 *Pten*

Pten encodes a phosphatase that antagonizes both PI3K/AKT and MAPK signaling cascades through its dual phosphatase activities (Myers et al., 1997). Thus, PTEN is a key element of the KIT/KITLG pathway. Interestingly, PTEN regulates its own expression by stabilizing its transcriptional activator TRP53 (Tang & Eng, 2006).

In the testis, PTEN is expressed in PGCs, but not in Sertoli cells (Kimura et al., 2003). Loss of PTEN leads to embryonic death, and heterozygotes have a high tumor incidence (Di Cristofano et al., 1998). PGCs lacking PTEN have defects in mitotic arrest and slow pluripotency loss after E13.5 (Fig. 1), and form EC clusters (Kimura et al., 2003). A high apoptotic rate is observed in the testis after E13.5 but remains insufficient to counterbalance abnormal proliferation. All mutant males develop bilateral TGCTs (Kimura et al., 2003). *Pten* transcript levels are reduced at least 2-fold in E13.5 gonads in MOLF males compared with 129 males (R. Zhu et al., 2007), suggesting that *Pten* is one of the genes on chromosome 19 that contribute to the high TGCT frequency. Furthermore, *Pten* is the only genetic variant that increases TGCT susceptibility to 100% in a mixed genetic background (Kimura et al., 2003).

Adenosine triphosphate-binding domains on PTEN regulate its subcellular localization (Lobo et al., 2009). Defect in these domains results in a predominantly nuclear localization, a DNA repair defect, and an inappropriate regulation of G1/S progression associated with a reduced apoptotic rate (He et al., 2011). PTEN mislocalization also leads to a reduced nuclear TRP53 level and transcriptional activity (He et al., 2011). Thus, PTEN plays an important role in cell growth and tumorigenesis, by regulating apoptosis, pluripotency, chromosome stability, DNA repair and cell cycle arrest (Kimura et al., 2003; Shen et al., 2007; Saal et al., 2008; He et al., 2011). Whether PTEN localization affects TGCT susceptibility is an open question.

3.3 *Trp53*

The *Trp53* gene encodes a tumor suppressor expressed in both PGCs and pre-Sertoli cells during embryogenesis, down-regulated after the birth in spermatogonia, and re-expressed in primary spermatocytes at pachytene, suggesting a role for TRP53 in control of meiosis (Almon et al., 1993; Schwartz et al., 1993). TRP53 activity is under the control of the PI3K/AKT pathway and depends of TRP53 phosphorylation (Xu, 2003). TRP53 regulates expression of several genes encoding mitotic regulators (i.e. CDKN1a, cyclin G1), the tumor suppressor PTEN, the pluripotent factor NANOG, and several apoptotic regulators (i.e. BAX, NOXA, PUMA) (Lin et al., 2005; Michalak et al., 2005; Tang & Eng, 2006). TRP53 also activates PUMA, which controls activity of BCL2 components and induces a mitochondria-dependent apoptosis (Chipuk et al., 2004; D. Liu et al., 2010). Thus, TRP53 controls many key cellular pathways including apoptosis, pluripotency, G1/S cell cycle arrest, and meiosis.

DNA damage leads to deficiency of both germ and Sertoli cells after γ-irradiation of fetal testis due to apoptosis and a proliferation defect (Lambrot et al., 2007). PGC deficiency is associated with increased TRP53 activity and induction of *BAX*, *PUMA* and *CDKN1a* expression (Lambrot et al., 2007). In mice, loss of TRP53 phosphorylation leads to constitutive activation of TRP53 and in turn too embryonic lethality (D. Liu et al., 2010). In contrast, *Trp53* -/- mice have normal development but a significantly reduced lifespan due to high predisposition for spontaneous tumors, especially lymphomas (Donehower et al., 1992; Jacks et al., 1994). Disruption of the *Trp53* gene in a pure 129 background increases TGCT incidence to 35-50% (Fig. 1) (Rotter et al., 1993; Donehower et al., 1995). Homozygotes have a giant-cell degenerative syndrome characterized by abnormal primary spermatocytes that arrest meiosis at pachytene, and form clusters leading to germ cell deficiency but remain fertile (Rotter et al., 1993). Heterozygotes are fertile with a 2-fold increase of TGCT frequency in the 129 strain (Rotter et al., 1993; Donehower et al., 1995). In a 50/50 mixed background of C57BL/6 and 129, the TGCT incidence is reduced to ~20% (Jacks et al., 1994). On these backgrounds, heterozygotes exhibit apparently normal testicular morphology (Rotter et al., 1993; Jacks et al., 1994; Muller et al., 2000). Thus, the combination of the *Trp53* defect and the 129 genetic background results in a synergistic increase of giant-cell syndrome and TGCT penetrance.

3.4 *Dmrt1*

Dmrt1 encodes a male-specific transcriptional factor (Raymond et al., 1999). In the testis, DMRT1 is strongly expressed in pre-Sertoli cells and then in both Sertoli and undifferentiated germ cells from P1 onward (Raymond et al., 1999). DMRT1 disappears in germ cells that enter meiosis, suggesting that DMRT1 regulates initiation of either meiosis, mitotic arrest, or both, in a stage-dependent manner (Raymond et al., 2000; Fahrioglu et al., 2007). During embryogenesis, DMRT1 controls transformation of PGCs into gonocytes by regulating expression of pluripotent factors such as SOX2 and NANOG, and their entrance into a quiescent state by controlling some cell cycle inhibitors such as CDKN2d (Krentz et al., 2009; Murphy et al., 2010). After birth, the DMRT1 control of cell cycle kinases allows mitotic reactivation of male gonocytes. DMRT1 also plays a role in radial migration (Fahrioglu et al., 2007). Finally, DMRT1 acts as a transcriptional gatekeeper that controls the switch from mitosis to meiosis in the undifferentiated spermatogonia (Matson et al., 2010).

Interestingly, DMRT1 also has an indirect control of critical developmental steps by regulating expression of the retinaldehyde dehydrogenases ALDH1A1 and ADH4 (Matson et al., 2010). These enzymes are expressed in Sertoli cells and convert vitamin A-derived retinal into retinoic acid. Retinoic acid regulates cell proliferation, migration and differentiation (Bowles et al., 2006; Koubova et al., 2006). Catabolism of retinoic acid is facilitated by cytochrome P450 enzymes such as CYP26B1, which is highly expressed until E13.5 by mitochondria in Sertoli cells (Li et al., 2009). Moreover, retinoic acid signaling is under the control of NANOS2, which is an RNA binding protein located in P-bodies, and is essential for male PGC development (Tsuda et al., 2003; A. Suzuki & Saga, 2008). PGCs lacking CYP26B1 enter meiosis at E13.5 and have a high apoptotic rate (MacLean et al.,

2007). Similarly, NANOS2 loss affects gonocytes that re-enter in the proliferative phase at E15, immediately initiate meiosis, and finally are completely depleted at E18.5 (Tsuda et al., 2003; A. Suzuki & Saga, 2008). DMRT1 loss in the 129 strain increases 10-fold the numbers of PGCs that escape mitotic arrest at E16.5 and return into pluripotent state to form EC clusters but without re-entry into meiosis as observed in *Nanos2* $^{-/-}$ and *Cyp26b1* $^{-/-}$ mutants (Raymond et al., 2000; Krentz et al., 2009). Thus, NANOS2, CYP26B1 and consequently retinoic acid are required in PGCs for quiescence, meiosis and survival, whereas DMRT1 is only required for quiescence and differentiation despite its role on retinoic acid pathway. Furthermore, *Dmrt1*$^{-/-}$ males are sterile and 90% of those develop TGCTs (Fig. 1) (Krentz et al., 2009). Interestingly, heterozygotes are fertile and the incidence of TGCTs is similar to that in 129 wild-type mice, suggesting that DMRT1 is haplo-insufficient for TGCTs.

3.5 *A^y* and *Eif2s2*

The *Agouti-yellow* (*A^y*), which is a ~170 kb deletion on chromosome 2 in mice includes the entire coding region of both *Eif2s2* and *Raly* genes as well as a part of the *Agouti* gene (Michaud et al., 1994). *Eif2s2* gene encodes the beta subunit of translation initiation factor eIF2 (Sarre, 1989). *Raly* encodes an RNA-binding protein that acts in pre-mRNA processing. *Agouti* encodes a signaling protein involved in the pigment synthesis in melanocytes (Michaud et al., 1994). Interestingly, the *A^y* deletion places the coding region of *Agouti* under the control of the *Raly* promoter, resulting in ectopic expression of *Agouti* (Duhl et al., 1994). As a result, *Agouti* is expressed in both PGCs and Sertoli cells, while RALY and eIF2s2 are lost in embryonic testes of A^y mice (Heaney et al., 2009). Homozygosity for *A^y* results in a pre-implantation lethality, whereas heterozygous *A^y* mice develop obesity, diabetes, yellow coat color traits, and have an increase of the propensity to develop a variety of spontaneous tumors (Duhl et al., 1994). Surprisingly, the *A^y* allele is the only genetic modifier known to suppress TGCT susceptibility in 129 mice and this phenotype results from loss of *Eif2s2* (Lam et al., 2004; Heaney et al., 2009). Indeed, loss of one *Eif2s2* allele decreases at least 2-fold (less for *A^y* allele) the high TGCT susceptibility observed in the 129-M19/M19 males (Fig. 1) (Lam et al., 2004; Heaney et al., 2009). This protective effect is due to a rescue of the G1/S mitotic arrest from E16.5 onward, but without effect on apoptosis, suggesting that *Eif2s2* deficiency affects only the mitotic activity but not the survival of PGCs (Heaney et al., 2009). In addition, spermatogenesis is normal in the mutant adult testis although the weight of testes is significantly reduced compared with their control 129-M19/M19 males, suggesting that reduced *Eif2s2* impedes but does not repress adult germ cell maturation (Heaney et al., 2009).

By using genetic targeting in mice, several genes have been identified that play a crucial role in PGC development and transformation into TGCTs. These genes act in distinct pathways and understanding their interrelation is a challenge for future research.

4. From mouse models to humans: Molecular basis of TGCT development

In this section, we compare results for genetic studies of TGCT susceptibility in humans and in mice (Table 1), with an emphasis on gene functions and protein pathways that control development of the PGC stem cell lineage and that modulate susceptibility to TGCTs.

4.1 The KIT/KITLG pathway

The KIT/KITLG pathway controls migration, proliferation, survival and differentiation of PGCs during embryogenesis and spermatogenesis. Although both *Kit* and *Kitlg* mutations affect development of several stem cell lineages including PGCs, only specific mutations in the *Kitlg* gene affect TGCT risk in mice (Heaney et al., 2008). In humans, four different GWAS identified allelic variations at the *KITLG* locus in individuals with TGCTs (Rapley et al., 2009; Turnbull et al., 2010; Kanetsky et al., 2009, 2011). Somatic mutations of *KIT* are also reported in men with TGCTs (Looijenga et al., 2003). In addition, deregulated expression of KITLG and KIT was found in TGCT biopsies (Murty et al., 1992). Thus, the KIT/KITLG pathway appears to be crucial for TGCT development both in humans and mice.

Similar evidence supports the hypothesis that the PI3K/AKT and MAPK signaling cascades modulate PGC transformation into TGCTs in humans and in mice:

- The *SPROUTY 4 (SPRY4)* gene encodes an inhibitor of MAPK signaling by inhibiting RAS activation (Leeksma et al., 2002). *SPRY4* is associated with TGCT susceptibility in humans (Rapley et al., 2009; Turnbull et al., 2010; Kanetsky et al., 2009, 2011).
- TRP53 deficiency is a potent but unusual modifier of TGCT susceptibility in both humans and mice. Although common in many cancers in humans (K. Suzuki & Matsubara, 2011), somatic *TRP53* mutations are exceptionally rare in TGCTs in humans (Murty et al., 1994; Peng et al., 1995); somatic *Trp53* mutations do not appear to have been surveyed in mice. By contrast, germline *TRP53* mutations are the molecular basis for Li-Fraumeni syndrome, which increases susceptibility to various cancers including TGCTs (Malkin et al., 1990), and germline *Trp53* mutations also increase susceptibility to many cancers including TGCTs in mice (Rotter et al., 1993; Donehower et al., 1995). Together these observations suggest that *TRP53* mutations act in the soma, rather than in the germline, to promote transformation of PGCs.

Various elements of TRP53-mediated apoptosis have been implicated in TGCT development. Indeed, variation within the *BAK1* gene is associated with TGCT cases in humans (Rapley et al., 2009; Turnbull et al., 2010). In addition, expression of *Cox15*, which encodes the mitochondrial cytochrome C oxidase assembly protein that is essential for the cell death program, is altered in testes of 129-M19 mice, which have a dramatically elevated TGCT risk (R. Zhu et al., 2007).

Interestingly, double homozygosity for the *KITLG* and *DMRT1* risk haplotypes increases risk 14-fold in humans (Kanetsky et al., 2011), suggesting that these haplotypes affect TGCTs in a non-additive manner. These interactions could arise either through pathways downstream of KIT that regulate DMRT1 activity, or through membrane-bound KITLG activating an intrinsic pathway in Sertoli cells that modulate the DMRT1 or the retinoic acid pathways. Pre-Sertoli cells are depleted in *Kitlg*^{Sl} mutants (Tajima et al., 1991) and their development is altered in *Dmrt1* -/- mice (Raymond et al., 2000; Krentz et al., 2009), suggesting that DMRT1 and KITLG are essential to Sertoli cell development and that pre-Sertoli cells might be involved in tumorigenesis, reinforcing the hypothesis of functional relations between KIT/KITLG and DMRT1. Finally, it is possible that at least one element of the KIT/KITLG pathway is a target gene of the transcriptional regulator DMRT1.

Chromosome #	QTL	Location human	Location mouse	Gene	Reference human	Reference mouse
2	D2S171	2p23	12A1	DNMT3A ?	Crockford et al., 2006	
3	D3S1607-D3S1282	3q26	3F2	TERC	Crockford et al., 2006	
4	rs4699052	4q24	3G3	CENP-E ?	Rapley et al., 2009	
	Somatic mutations	4q12	5C3	KIT	Looijenga et al., 2003	
5	rs4624820	5q31	18B3	SPRY4	Rapley et al., 2009 Kanetsky et al., 2009, 2011 Turnbull et al., 2010	
		5q31	18B2	DND1		Noguchi & Noguchi, 1985 Youngren et al., 2005
		5q31	18B2	PAIP2 ?		Asada et al., 1994
	rs2736100 rs4635969	5p15	13C1	TERT	Turnbull et al., 2010	
6	rs210138	6p21	17A3	BAK1	Rapley et al., 2009 Turnbull et al., 2010	
9	rs755383 rs7040024	9p24	19B	DMRT1	Turnbull et al., 2010 Kanetsky et al., 2011	Youngren et al., 2003 Krentz et al., 2009
		9q24	19C1	SMARCA2 ?		Youngren et al., 2003
10		10p11	18A1	MAP3K8 ?		Anderson et al., 2009a
		10q23	19C1	PTEN		Kimura et al., 2003
		10q24	19C3	COX15?		R. Zhu et al., 2007
		10q25	19D2	GFRA1 ?		Matin et al., 2000 Youngren et al., 2003
		10q26	19D3	NANOS1 ? EIF3a ?		Matin et al., 2000 Youngren et al., 2003
12	rs995030 rs4474514 rs1508595	12q21	10D1	KITLG	Rapley et al., 2009 Kanetsky et al., 2009, 2011 Turnbull et al., 2010	McCoshen & McCallion, 1975 Copeland et al., 1990 Heaney et al., 2008
	D12S85-D12S368	12q13	(15F1?)	HDAC7? DDX23?	Crockford et al., 2006	
	rs2900333	12p13	6G1	ATF7IP	Turnbull et al., 2010	
17		17p13	11B13	TRP53		Donehower et al., 1995 Rotter et al., 1993
18	D18S5	18q22	18E4	DOK6 ?	Murty et al., 1994 Crockford et al., 2006	
		18q21	18E2	MBD1/MBD2, MAPK4 ?		Anderson et al., 2009a
20		20q11	2H1	EIF2s2		Heaney et al., 2009
21		21q22	10C1	DNMT3L	Minami et al., 2010	
X	*Tgct1* locus	Xq27	(12C1?)	SPANX ?	Rapley et al., 2000 Crockford et al., 2006	Hammond et al., 2007
	DXS548 - DXS8091	Xq27	XA7	FMR1 ?	Crockford et al., 2006	
		Xq28	XA7	DKC1 ?	Skotheim et al., 2001	
Y	gr/gr deletion	Yq11	?	DAZ, BPY2, CDY1	Nathanson et al., 2005	Anderson et al., 2009b
		Yp11	YA1	TSPY	Y.F. Lau, 1999 Akimoto et al., 2010	

Table 1. Candidate modifiers of TGCTs in humans and their orthologues in mice.

Other tyrosine kinase receptors that are expressed in PGCs may also contribute to TGCT development. A strong candidate is RET, which is activated by the growth factor GDNF receptor GFRA1. *Gfra1* gene is located at 19D3 in mice, within a locus that was proposed as candidate TGCT modifier (Matin et al., 1999; Youngren et al., 2003). Furthermore, *Ret* is a known proto-oncogene (Grieco et al., 1990) and its expression is indirectly under the control of the TGCT modifier DMRT1 (Krentz et al., 2009). Allelic variations were identified at 18q21 in TGCTs in humans (Murty et al., 1994; Crockford et al., 2006). This locus contains the *Docking protein 6* (*DOK6*) gene that plays a role in RET signaling cascade (Crowder et al., 2004). Interestingly, *Dok6* gene is located on chromosome 18 in mice, reinforcing the hypothesis of the role of other tyrosine kinase receptors such as GDNF receptors on TGCT development (Anderson et al., 2009a).

4.2 Telomerase and TGCTs

By extending the TTAGGG telomeric nucleotide repeats, telomerase counterbalances loss of telomere length that usually occurs during cell division, and thus preserves chromosomal integrity (Venteicher et al., 2009). The active telomerase complex involves TERT (telomerase inverse transcriptase), the RNA component TERC, the ribonucleoprotein dyskerin (encoded by the X-linked *DCK1* gene) and several other cofactors (Venteicher et al., 2009). Telomerase is activated by the telomerase Cajal body protein-1 (TCAB1) which is encoded by the *WRAP53* gene (Jady et al., 2004).

Mutations in *TERT* (Marrone et al., 2007), *TERC* (Vulliamy et al., 2001), *DKC1* (Heiss et al., 1998) and more recently *WRAP53* (Zhong et al., 2011), which all lead to absence or dysfunction of telomerase, are found in congenital dyskeratosis, a human genetic deficiency characterized by abnormal skin pigmentation, bone marrow failure, and an elevated tumor frequency. Telomere defects are also associated with segmental progeria syndrome, which is characterized by accelerated ageing and is associated with a severe deficiency of adult stem cells in brain, bone marrow and testis (Burtner & Kennedy, 2010). Furthermore, telomerase dysfunction enhances tumor incidence in mice (Blasco et al., 1997). Thus, telomerase seems to play an essential role in stem cell development and cancer formation.

Specific markers of TGCT susceptibility have been recently identified in humans at 12p13, which contains the gene encoding ATF7IP, an enhancer of *TERT* and *TERC* transcription, and at 5p15 within *TERT* (Turnbull et al., 2010). Furthermore, a marker of familial TGCT risk was located 50kb downstream of *TERC* (Crockford et al., 2006), and amplification of human Xq28 containing *DCK1* was found in TGCTs (Skotheim et al., 2001). In mice, the *primordial germ cell tumor 1* locus (*pgct1*), that contains *Tert* on chromosome 13, has been identified as an enhancer of TGCT susceptibility (Muller et al., 2000). Furthermore, loss of *Tert* in mice leads to PGC deficiency which increases accross generations, due to both reduced proliferation and increased apoptosis (Lee et al., 1998). This phenotype is more severe in males where PGC deficiency is complete at the sixth generation (Lee et al., 1998). Taking together, these observations highlight the involvement of telomerase and telomere biology in TGCT development.

Interestingly, *pgct1* locus interacts with TRP53 to modulate TGCT susceptibility in mice (Muller et al., 2000), and *Wrap53* is a natural antisense transcript of *Trp53* and regulates the levels of TRP53 in response to DNA damage (Mahmoudi et al., 2009). Furthermore, telomerase dysfunction activates TRP53-dependent apoptosis (Chin et al., 1999). By contrast, progeria-like syndromes have been associated with alterations in TRP53-dependent apoptosis (D. Liu et al., 2010). Given these results and that both congenital dyskeratosis and segmental progeria affect similar stem cell lineages as KIT/KITLG defect (melanogenesis, gametogenesis and hematopoiesis), we propose an interrelation between KIT/KITLG pathway, via *TRP53*, and telomerase, via *TERT* and *WRAP53*, during embryogenesis that contributes to tumorigenesis.

4.3 Sex chromosomes and TGCTs

Males with Klinefelter's syndrome (also known as XXY syndrome) have 50-fold greater TGCT risk (Gustavson et al., 1975). Secondly, gain of X chromosomes has been described in TGCTs in humans (Peltomaki et al., 1990; Skotheim et al., 2001). Third, chromosome X from the C57BL/6 strain reduces tumor incidence in 129-*Ter/Ter* mice (Hammond et al., 2007), suggesting that genes linked to chromosome X both in mice and humans modulate TGCT incidence. In addition to *DCK1* at Xq28 in humans, other interesting genes are *Sperm protein associated with the nucleus mapped to the X chromosome* (*SpanX*) clusters at Xq27, a locus named *Tgct1*, which has been linked with bilateral TGCTs and undescended testicular syndrome in humans (Rapley et al., 2000; Kouprina et al., 2004; Crockford et al., 2006). Although the function of SPANX proteins is unknown, evidence is accumulating that suggests their involvement in tumorigenesis. For example, *SPANX* genes are deregulated in Down's syndrome subjects who have undescended testis and an increased risk of TGCTs (Satge et al., 1997), further suggesting interaction of genes located on chromosome X and chromosome 21 for TGCT susceptibility. *SPANX* genes have a testis-specific expression that is conserved in rodents and humans, and was also detected in EC clusters and TGCTs (Westbrook et al., 2004; Salemi et al., 2006).

Similarly, a complete loss of chromosome Y in humans (45 XO karyotype) reduces TGCT susceptibility (Soh et al., 1992). Furthermore, the rare *gr/gr* deletion of the Y chromosome that removes part of the AZFc region (Yq11) is found in men with infertility and low-penetrance for TGCT susceptibility (Nathanson et al., 2005). This deletion affects *DAZ* (deleted in azoospermia), *BPY2* (Basic protein, Y-linked) and *CDY1* (chromodomain protein, Y-linked 1). *DAZ* encodes an RNA-binding protein that interacts with the P-body component PUM2 in PGCs (Moore et al., 2003). The functions of CDY1 and BPY2 remain unknown. Moreover, aberrant expression of *testis-specific protein on Y* (TSPY) at Yp11 in humans may contribute to predisposition for TGCTs (Y.F. Lau, 1999), revealing a differential effect of the Y chromosome on TGCT risk. In mice, neither the MOLF-derived nor the C57BL/6-derived chromosome Y significantly affects susceptibility in 129 mice (Hammond et al., 2007). However, by using a sex-reversed mouse model, TGCTs were not found in the absence of the Y chromosome (Anderson et al., 2009b). Furthermore, a possible interaction, which suppress TGCT susceptibility in mice, was described between the Y-linked genes, which have a low-penetrance for TGCTs, and either the *Dnd1* gene (chromosome 18) or the genes located on chromosome 19 (perhaps *Dmrt1* given its role in sex differentiation and in TGCT susceptibility) (Anderson et al., 2009b). This hypothesis is supported by the fact that *Dnd1* has sex-dependent effects on PGC survival and tumor susceptibility. Indeed, *Dnd1* is differentially expressed in XX (down-regulation) and XY (up-regulation) gonads (Youngren et al., 2005). Loss of *Dnd1* leads to PGC deficiency that increases with age in males, but not in females (T. Noguchi & M. Noguchi, 1985). Furthermore, the few mutant germ cells that successfully migrate to the gonad give rise to mature oocytes in females, while in testes, they give rise to TGCTs in 95% of cases (Cook et al., 2009).

Thus, sex chromosomes seem to play a crucial role in TGCT susceptibility. Identification of the candidate genes and of their interrelation remains to be elucidated.

4.4 RNA biology, epigenetic regulation and TGCTs

The translational complex eIF2 is composed of the alpha (eIF2s1), beta (eIF2s2) and gamma (eIF2s3) subunits (Sarre, 1989). *Eif2s2* is a TGCT modifier in mice (Heaney et al., 2009), but remains to be confirmed in humans. *Eif2s3* is located on both Y (*Eif2s3y*) and X (*Eif2s3x*) chromosomes in mice (in humans, no Y homologues have been found) (Ehrmann et al., 1998). Given the role of sex chromosomes discussed above, *Eif2s3* should be considered as a candidate for TGCT susceptibility. EIF4E is another translational factor which acts downstream of PI3K/AKT pathway. Interestingly, eIF4E is a potent oncogene (Wendel et al., 2004), regulated by the poly(A)-binding protein and its cofactor PAIP2 (Yanagiya et al., 2010). *Paip2* is located on mouse chromosome 18 near the *Ter* locus (Asada et al., 1994). Finally, *Eif3a* encodes another translational factor located on chromosome 19 in mice within a region involved in TGCT susceptibility (Matin et al., 1999; Youngren et al., 2003), but its direct role in TGCTs remains to be tested in mice and humans.

Translation is under the control of P-bodies, which regulate many mRNA processes (i.e. post-transcriptional regulation, degradation, storage, transport, and stabilization) in cells under normal physiological conditions or in response to stress (Seydoux & Braun, 2006; Parker & Sheth, 2007). P-bodies are essential for male PGC development and probably also for tumorigenesis given the involvement of its major components (Hayashi et al., 2008; K.M. Nelson & Weiss, 2008). *DDX3,* which encodes a helicase of P-body, is located on both Y (*DDX3y*) and X (*DDX3x*) chromosomes in mice and humans, and has been identified as a tumor suppressor (Chao et al., 2006). Given the role of sex chromosomes and the close location of *Ddx3y* and *Eif2s3y* in mice, *DDX3* should also be considered as a candidate for TGCT susceptibility. Interestingly, another *DDX* gene (*DDX23*) is located at 12q13 in humans, a locus which has been associated with TGCTs (Crockford et al., 2006). In addition, PGCs lacking DICER1, another helicase, are depleted around E13.5 in mice (Hayashi et al., 2008), suggesting an essential role of *Dicer1* in PGC development. *Dicer1* has been also identified as a potential tumor suppressor in mice and probably also in humans (Su et al., 2010). *Nanos1,* which encodes an RNA binding protein, is located on chromosome 19 in mice, within a region involved in TGCT susceptibility (Matin et al., 1999; Youngren et al., 2003). Finally, allelic variations within the *X-fragile mental retardation* (*FMR*) genes (*FMR1, FMR1nb* and *FMR2*) at Xq27 in humans have been identified in TGCTs (Crockford et al., 2006). These genes encode RNA binding proteins that are involved in translation regulation through an interaction with the DICER and Argonaute proteins (Jin et al., 2004). The number of CGG trinucleotide repeats in the 5′-untranslated region of *FMR1* and their DNA methylation pattern determine the severity of FMR-related pathogenicity (Fu et al., 1991; McConkie-Rosell et al., 1993). Furthermore, loss of *Fmr1* alters both proliferation and differentiation of several stem cell lineages including PGCs (Castren et al., 2005), suggesting a role of *FMR1* in TGCT susceptibility.

Additional evidence shows an association between DNA methylation and TGCT susceptibility. First, DNA methylation in male PGCs is largely erased at E10.5-E11.5 and partially reestablished at E13-E14 (Sasaki & Matsui, 2008). This epigenetic reprogramming completely overlaps the critical period for TGCT formation (E11.5-E13.5) (Stevens & Little, 1954; Stevens, 1967). Secondly, the DNA methyltransferase DNMT3L has been recently identified as a novel marker of TGCTs in humans (Minami et al., 2010), in accordance with the fact that TGCTs have a distinct epigenetic profile from other cancers (Ushida et al., 2011). Third, other genetic markers for TGCTs have been identified: (1) in humans, at 2p23 which contains *DNMT3A*, and at 12q13 which contains gene encoding the histone deacetylase HDAC7 (Crockford et al., 2006); (2) in mice, on a region of chromosome 18 that contains genes encoding two methyl-binding proteins MBD1 and MBD2 (Anderson et al., 2009a), and on chromosome 19 at a region that contains the remodeling chromatin factor *Smarca2* (Matin et al., 1999; Youngren et al., 2003). Other studies correlate up-regulation of DNMT3A with demethylation of specific loci in TGCTs in humans (Ishii et al., 2007), and inhibition of both DNMTs and HDACs with prevention of cancer formation (W.G. Zhu & Otterson, 2003). Another TGCT marker has been identified at 4q24 in humans near the *CENP-E* gene that encodes a centromeric-associated protein required for establishing and maintaining of the mitotic checkpoint (Abrieu et al., 2000; Rapley et al., 2009). CENP-E is described in mice as tumor-suppressing or -promoting factor depending on the context (Weaver et al., 2007). Interestingly, TRP53 has been associated with DNA demethylation (Ashur-Fabian et al., 2010) and several TRP53-target genes show aberrant methylation pattern in TGCTs in humans (Christoph et al., 2007).

5. Transgenerational genetic effects on TGCT susceptibility

Growing evidence suggests an alternative molecular basis of inheritance that complements conventional Mendelian inheritance with a similar strength, frequency and persistence across multiple generations (V.R. Nelson & Nadeau, 2010). These alternatives could involve four different forms: (1) environmental factors that create an epigenetic state that persists across generations (transgenerational environmental effects); (2) ancestral genetic factors that are sufficient to initiate epigenetic inheritance (transgenerational genetic effects); (3) environmental factors that have an epigenetic effect only in genetically predisposed individuals (transgenerational gene-environmental interactions); and (4) genetic variants in parents and others in offspring that interact to create an epigenetic state in offspring (transgenerational gene-gene interactions) (V.R. Nelson & Nadeau, 2010). The evidence for transgenerational genetic effects, as well as the implication inheritance of TGCT susceptibility will be discussed in this section.

5.1 Environmental effects

Pesticides and insecticides were intensively used in agricultural industries during previous decades. These chemicals, which are now found in foods and water, contain endocrine disruptors that act primarily through nuclear hormone receptors such as estrogen and androgen receptors (Danchin et al., 2011). *In utero*, perinatal or neonatal exposures affect male reproduction leading to infertility with an increase of testicular abnormalities and germ cell cancers in humans (A. Giwercman & Y.L. Giwercman, 2011). These effects can be reversible, permanent or even transgenerational, and involve alterations of DNA methylation (Anway et al., 2005; Danchin et al., 2011; Kalfa et al., 2011).

Other natural nutrients could also modulate predisposition to disease such as TGCTs. As discussed above, vitamin A plays an essential role in PGC development and might also influence TGCT susceptibility. Similarly, folate which is a methyl-donor nutrient affects DNA methylation and is essential for PGC development (Danchin et al., 2011). Determining the effects of folate and vitamins on TGCT susceptibility, and whether supply of these nutrients can reverse TGCT development is a challenge for future research both in rodents and humans. A related challenge is understanding relation between genetic modifiers and environmental factors on TGCT susceptibility.

5.2 Parent-of-origin effects

While environmental factors could affect reproductive health across generations in a parent-of-origin manner (Anway et al., 2005; Kalfa et al., 2011), two examples reveal similar parental-dependent transgenerational effect of TGCT modifier genes in mice.

Loss of KITLG (*Kitlg*^{Sl}, *Kitlg*^{SlJ} and *Kitlg*^{Slgb}) in mice causes 2-fold increase of TGCT susceptibility in the 129 strain (Stevens, 1967; Heaney et al., 2008). Surprisingly, among the progeny of the *Kitlg*^{Slgb}/+ males, wild-type sons never develop TGCTs (5% expected), whereas wild-type sons of the reciprocal crosses (maternal *Kitlg*^{Slgb} allele) are affected at the expected rate (Fig. 2) (Heaney et al., 2008). Thus, absence of one *Kitlg* allele in the male germline leads to an epigenetic change that affects TGCT susceptibility in the predisposed 129 strain. Whether this protective effect persists across generations is currently being tested (E. Leung & J.H. Nadeau). Determining the molecular basis of this epigenetic modification, and whether other *Kitlg* mutant males (i.e. *Kitlg*^{Sl} and *Kitlg*^{SlJ}) have similar effects remain to be determined.

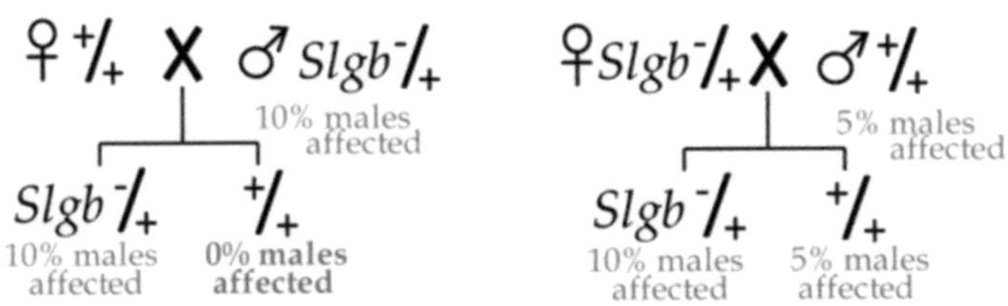

Fig. 2. Example of parental transgenerational effects in a mouse model for TGCTs.

Similarly, wild-type sons of females with the *A*^{y} allele, which acts as a TGCT suppressor due to the deletion of *Eif2s2*, have a 65% of risk being affected (80% expected) (Heaney et al., 2009; J.D. Heaney & J.H. Nadeau, unpublished), revealing another example of a transgenerational effect on TGCTs transmitted in this case through the maternal germ-lineage.

5.3 Gene-gene interactions

The intercross of *Trp53* -/+ and *Kit*^{Wv} -/+ mice yields {*Kit*^{Wv} -/+; *Trp53* -/+} double heterozygotes which are intercrossed to generate double homozygotes (Jordan et al., 1999). Surprisingly, {*Kit*^{Wv} -/-; *Trp53* -/-} males are fertile due to a rescue of PGCs at E13.5 (Jordan et al., 1999), confirming that the high rate of apoptosis observed in *Kit*^{Wv} -/- embryonic gonads depends on KIT/KITLG-TRP53 interactions. Loss of both TRP53 alleles is necessary to rescue fertility because both {*Kit*^{Wv} $^{-}/_{-}$; *Trp53* $^{+}/_{+}$} and {*Kit*^{Wv} $^{-}/_{-}$; *Trp53* $^{-}/_{+}$} males are sterile (Jordan et al., 1999). Interestingly, only 10% of normal {*Kit*^{Wv} $^{-}/_{-}$; *Trp53* $^{-}/_{-}$} germ cells are present in the adult testes, compared to 34% after birth. This deficiency in the adult testes correlates with presence of testicular abnormalities (germ cell radial migratory defect, meiotic failure and apoptosis). As discussed above, these testicular abnormalities could be the origin of TGCTs. Unfortunately, this study was conducted on a mixed background and the TGCT susceptibility of these offspring remains to be investigated in the 129 strain. However, intercrosses of *Trp53* $^{-}/_{+}$ and *Kitlg*^{SlJ} $^{-}/_{+}$ mice give the double heterozygous {*Kitlg*^{SlJ} $^{-}/_{+}$; *Trp53* $^{-}/_{+}$} males that have a surprising 4-fold reduced TGCT frequency (7%; 26% expected) (Lam et al., 2004), suggesting that *Kitlg* and *Trp53* genes can interact to counterbalance their effects on TGCT susceptibility. The effect of this gene interaction on PGC development remains to be investigated.

Kitlg^{SlJ} allele interacts also with the MOLF-derived chromosome 19. Indeed, the double heterozygotes {*Kitlg*^{SlJ} $^{-}/_{+}$; M19/$_{+}$} have a significantly increased TGCT susceptibility (57%; 45% expected) due to an increase in the number of bilateral cases (Lam et al., 2004). These results suggest that *Kitlg*^{SlJ} hemizygosity potentiates the effect of M19 on TGCT susceptibility.

The intercross of C57BL/6-*Bax* $^{-}/_{-}$ and 129-*Ter/Ter* mice yields double homozygotes {*Ter/Ter*; *Bax* $^{-}/_{-}$} that show at least 50% of PGCs rescued at E13.5 (Cook et al., 2009), demonstrating that the PGC deficiency in 129-*Ter/Ter* males is due to BAX-mediated apoptosis. However, rescued PGCs are completely lost in adult, suggesting that mechanisms affecting PGC development after E13 are BAX-independent in 129-*Ter/Ter* mice. This hypothesis is supported by the observation that loss of BAX does not affect the TGCT frequency, which remains elevated (91%; 94% expected) (Cook et al., 2009). Surprisingly, the {*Ter/Ter*; *Bax* $^{-}/_{+}$} males have a 2-fold decrease of tumor risk and {*Ter/Ter*; *Bax* $^{+}/_{+}$} males do not develop TGCTs (Cook et al., 2009). This protective phenotype is interesting but we cannot determine whether it results from a genetic background effect (C57BL/6 vs 129) or from a genetic interaction (*Bax* vs *Dnd1*). Backcrosses of the double homozygotes {*Ter/Ter*; *Bax* $^{-}/_{-}$} to pure C57BL/6 background mice suppress the TGCT susceptibility (Cook et al., 2011), favoring a background effect on TGCT susceptibility.

The double {*Ter/Ter*; *Sf1* $^{-}/_{+}$} mutants in the 129 strain have a 2-fold reduction in risk due to a reduced frequency of bilateral tumors (R. Zhu et al., 2010). Despite this protective effect on TGCT formation, all mutant males are sterile due to a complete germ cell deficiency (R. Zhu et al., 2010). This phenotype is similar as those observed in the {*Ter/Ter*; *Bax* $^{-}/_{+}$} males suggesting a common pathway involving both SF1 and BAX on PGC deficiency in 129-*Ter/Ter* mice.

The interaction of *Ter* allele with the four risk alleles *Kitlg*^{SlJ}, mutated *Trp53*, M19 and *A*^{y} in the respective double heterozygous males increased TGCT susceptibility at least 2-fold in the 129 strain by enhancing the frequency of bilateral tumors (Lam et al., 2007). Surprisingly, all {*Ter*/$_{+}$; $^{+}/_{+}$} males of these four intercrosses also have a 2-fold increase in TGCT frequency, suggesting transgenerational epistasis that acts only in the presence of the *Ter* allele in the offspring generation. The mechanism underlying interactions with the *Ter* allele remains elusive, although the new role of DND1 in the micro-RNA biology (Kedde et al., 2007) may be one ways by which this transgenerational effect acts.

6. Conclusions

Mouse models of TGCTs have made major contributions to stem cell biology, developmental biology of the PGC lineage, and genetic and epigenetic studies of TGCT susceptibility.

The germ cell lineage, which has been termed the 'mother of all stem cells', carries DNA and other molecular features that together constitute our genetic and epigenetic heritage (Donovan, 1998). Controlling differentiation and proliferation of PGCs, which belong to the only lineage of cells that naturally show totipotency is therefore essential for maintaining their integrity. Many factors have been shown to affect molecular mechanisms regulating pluripotency versus differentiation, proliferation versus death, and migration versus stasis during normal PGC development (Pesce et al., 1993; Lin et al., 2005; Shen et al., 2007; Heaney et al., 2009; Murphy et al., 2010; Cook et al., 2011). In parallel, insights are beginning to emerge about the ways in which anomalies in these factors and processes lead to transformation (Rotter et al., 1993; Kimura et al., 2003; Youngren et al., 2005; Heaney et al., 2008; Krentz et al., 2009). Despite their fundamental relevance to understanding important aspects of human biology, these studies are obviously difficult to conduct in humans. Thus, studies of PGCs and their transformed derivatives in mice will likely remain relevant to our understanding of the genetics and developmental origins of TGCTs in humans.

Despite being a common cancer in young men (Buetow, 1995), with heritable TGCT risk among the highest of all cancers (Gilbert et al., 2011), the genetic control of inherited susceptibility has proven to be remarkably elusive. However, with the availability of complete panels of genetic markers, high-throughput assays, and increasingly rigorous analytical methods, both linkage analysis and GWAS have begun to yield results. The first breakthrough involved the gr/gr deletion on the X chromosome (Nathanson et al., 2005), followed more recently with GWAS evidence for *KITLG, SPRY4, DMRT1, TERT, BAK1* and *ATF7IP* as strong candidate susceptibility genes (Rapley et al., 2009; Turnbull et al., 2010; Kanetsky et al., 2009, 2011). The recent evidence for involvement of *KITLG* in humans was anticipated by corresponding evidence in mice involving mutations in the *Kitlg* gene (Heaney et al., 2008). The fact that some but not all *Kitlg* mutants affect susceptibility implies that allele-specific tests and structure-function studies will both be important to understand the ways in which *KITLG* variants affect TGCT susceptibility in humans.

More recently, heritable epigenetic changes have been shown to strongly influence TGCT risk in mouse models. In particular, TGCT modifier genes in the parental generation were shown to interact with the *Dnd1* modifier to increase both the number of affected males and the proportion of bilateral cases (Lam et al., 2007). Similar evidence for transgenerational genetic effects has also been reported for *Kitlg* mutants (Heaney et al., 2008). These and related discoveries suggest that heritable epigenetic changes might be as important as conventional genetic effects in controlling inherited TGCT risk, and might account for the substantial difference in risk between sons and brothers of cases (Hutter et al., 1967). Identifying the nature of these epigenetic factors, characterizing their molecular mechanisms, and testing their contribution to TGCT susceptibility in humans and in mice remain major challenges.

7. Acknowledgement

Preparation of this review was supported with funds from NCI CA75056 and NIH Pioneer Award DP-12560002

8. References

Abrieu, A.; Kahana, J.A.; Wood, K.W. & Cleveland, D.W. (2000). CENP-E as an essential component of the mitotic checkpoint in vitro. *Cell,* Vol.102, No.6, (September 2000), pp.817-826, ISSN 0092-8674

Albrecht, K.H. & Eicher, E.M. (2001). Evidence that Sry is expressed in pre-Sertoli cells and Sertoli and granulosa cells have a common precursor. *Dev Biol,* Vol.240, No.1, (December 2001), pp.92-107, ISSN 0012-1606

Almon, E.; Goldfinger, N.; Kapon, A.; Schwartz, D.; Levine, A.J. & Rotter, V. (1993). Testicular tissue-specific expression of the p53 suppressor gene. *Dev Biol,* Vol.156, No.1, (March 1993), pp.107-116, ISSN 0012-1606

Anderson, P.D.; Nelson, V.R.; Tesar, P.J. & Nadeau, J.H. (2009a). Genetic factors on mouse chromosome 18 affecting susceptibility to testicular germ cell tumors and permissiveness to embryonic stem cell derivation. *Cancer Res,* Vol.69, No.23, (December 2009), pp.9112-9117, ISSN 1538-7445

Anderson, P.D.; Lam, M.Y.; Poirier, C.; Bishop, C.E. & Nadeau, J.H. (2009b). The role of the mouse y chromosome on susceptibility to testicular germ cell tumors. *Cancer Res,* Vol.69, No.8, (April 2009), pp.3614-3618, ISSN 1538-7445

Anway, M.D.; Cupp, A.S.; Uzumcu, M. & Skinner, M.K. (2005). Epigenetic transgenerational actions of endocrine disruptors and male fertility. *Science,* Vol.308, No.5727, (June 2005), pp.1466-1469, ISSN 1095-9203

Asada, Y.; Varnum, D.S.; Frankel, W.N. & Nadeau, J.H. (1994). A mutation in the Ter gene causing increased susceptibility to testicular teratomas maps to mouse chromosome 18. *Nat Genet,* Vol.6, No.4, (April 1994), pp.363-368, ISSN 1061-4036

Ashur-Fabian, O.; Har-Zahav, A.; Shaish, A.; Wiener Amram, H.; Margalit, O.; Weizer-Stern, O.; Dominissini, D.; Harats, D.; Amariglio, N. & Rechavi, G. (2010). apoB and apobec1, two genes key to lipid metabolism, are transcriptionally regulated by p53. *Cell Cycle,* Vol.9, No.18, (September 2010), pp.3761-3770, ISSN 1551-4005

Bernstein, A.; Forrester, L.; Reith, A.D.; Dubreuil, P. & Rottapel, R. (1991). The murine W/c-kit and Steel loci and the control of hematopoiesis. *Semin Hematol,* Vol.28, No.2, (April 1991), pp.138 142, ISSN 0037-1963

Besmer, P.; Manova, K.; Duttlinger, R.; Huang, E.J.; Packer, A.; Gyssler, C. & Bachvarova, R.F. (1993). The kit-ligand (steel factor) and its receptor c-kit/W: pleiotropic roles in gametogenesis and melanogenesis. *Dev Suppl,* pp.125-137

Blasco, M.A.; Lee, H.W.; Hande, M.P.; Samper, E.; Lansdorp, P.M.; DePinho, R.A. & Greider, C.W. (1997). Telomere shortening and tumor formation by mouse cells lacking telomerase RNA. *Cell,* Vol.91, No.1, (October 1997), pp.25-34, ISSN 0092-8674

Bowles, J.; Knight, D.; Smith, C.; Wilhelm, D.; Richman, J.; Mamiya, S.; Yashiro, K.; Chawengsaksophak, K.; Wilson, M.J.; Rossant, J.; Hamada, H. & Koopman, P. (2006). Retinoid signaling determines germ cell fate in mice. *Science,* Vol.312, No.5773, (April 2006), pp.596-600, ISSN 1095-9203

Brannan, C.I.; Bedell, M.A.; Resnick, J.L.; Eppig, J.J.; Handel, M.A.; Williams, D.E.; Lyman, S.D.; Donovan, P.J.; Jenkins, N.A. & Copeland, N.G. (1992). Developmental abnormalities in Steel17H mice result from a splicing defect in the steel factor cytoplasmic tail. *Genes Dev,* Vol.6, No.10, (October 1992), pp.1832-1842, ISSN 0890-9369

Buetow, S.A. (1995). Epidemiology of testicular cancer. *Epidemiol Rev,* Vol.17, No.2, pp.433-449, ISSN 0193-936X

Burtner, C.R. & Kennedy, B.K. (2010). Progeria syndromes and ageing: what is the connection? *Nat Rev Mol Cell Biol,* Vol.11, No.8, (August 2010), pp.567-578, ISSN 1471-0080

Carson, W.E.; Haldar, S.; Baiocchi, R.A.; Croce, C.M. & Caligiuri, M.A. (1994). The c-kit ligand suppresses apoptosis of human natural killer cells through the upregulation of bcl-2. *Proc Natl Acad Sci U S A,* Vol.91, No.16, (August 1994), pp.7553-7557, ISSN 0027-8424

Castren, M.; Tervonen, T.; Karkkainen, V.; Heinonen, S.; Castren, E.; Larsson, K.; Bakker, C.E.; Oostra, B.A. & Akerman, K. (2005). Altered differentiation of neural stem cells in fragile X syndrome. *Proc Natl Acad Sci U S A,* Vol.102, No.49, (December 2005), pp.17834-17839, ISSN 0027-8424

Chao, C.H.; Chen, C.M.; Cheng, P.L.; Shih, J.W.; Tsou, A.P. & Lee, Y.H. (2006). DDX3, a DEAD box RNA helicase with tumor growth-suppressive property and transcriptional regulation activity of the p21waf1/cip1 promoter, is a candidate tumor suppressor. *Cancer Res,* Vol.66, No.13, (July 2006), pp.6579-6588, ISSN 0008-5472

Chin, L.; Artandi, S.E.; Shen, Q.; Tam, A.; Lee, S.L.; Gottlieb, G.J.; Greider, C.W. & DePinho, R.A. (1999). p53 deficiency rescues the adverse effects of telomere loss and cooperates with telomere dysfunction to accelerate carcinogenesis. *Cell,* Vol.97, No.4, (May 1999), pp.527-538, ISSN 0092-8674

Chipuk, J.E.; Kuwana, T.; Bouchier-Hayes, L.; Droin, N.M.; Newmeyer, D.D.; Schuler, M. & Green, D.R. (2004). Direct activation of Bax by p53 mediates mitochondrial membrane permeabilization and apoptosis. *Science,* Vol.303, No.5660, (Februar 2004), pp.1010-1014, ISSN 1095-9203

Christoph, F.; Kempkensteffen, C.; Weikert, S.; Krause, H.; Schostak, M.; Miller, K. & Schrader, M. (2007). Frequent epigenetic inactivation of p53 target genes in seminomatous and nonseminomatous germ cell tumors. *Cancer Lett,* Vol.247, No.1, (March 2007), pp.137-142, ISSN 0304-3835

Clark, J.M. & Eddy, E.M. (1975). Fine structural observations on the origin and associations of primordial germ cells of the mouse. *Dev Biol,* Vol.47, No.1, (November 1975), pp.136-155, ISSN 0012-1606

Cook, M.S.; Coveney, D.; Batchvarov, I.; Nadeau, J.H. & Capel, B. (2009). BAX-mediated cell death affects early germ cell loss and incidence of testicular teratomas in Dnd1(Ter/Ter) mice. *Dev Biol,* Vol.328, No.2, (April 2009), pp.377-383, ISSN 1095-564X

Cook, M.S.; Munger, S.C.; Nadeau, J.H. & Capel, B. (2011). Regulation of male germ cell cycle arrest and differentiation by DND1 is modulated by genetic background. *Development,* Vol.138, No.1, (January 2011), pp.23-32, ISSN 1477-9129

Copeland, N.G.; Gilbert, D.J.; Cho, B.C.; Donovan, P.J.; Jenkins, N.A.; Cosman, D.; Anderson, D.; Lyman, S.D. & Williams, D.E. (1990). Mast cell growth factor maps near the steel locus on mouse chromosome 10 and is deleted in a number of steel alleles. *Cell,* Vol.63, No.1, (October 1990), pp.175-183, ISSN 0092-8674

Copeland, N.G.; Jenkins, N.A.; Gilbert, D.J.; Eppig, J.T.; Maltais, L.J.; Miller, J.C.; Dietrich, W.F.; Weaver, A.; Lincoln, S.E.; Steen, R.G. et al. (1993). A genetic linkage map of the mouse: current applications and future prospects. *Science,* Vol.262, No.5130, (October 1993), pp.57-66, ISSN 0036-8075

Crockford, G.P.; Linger, R.; Hockley, S.; Dudakia, D.; Johnson, L.; Huddart, R.; Tucker, K.; Friedlander, M.; Phillips, K.A.; Hogg, D.; Jewett, M.A.; Lohynska, R.; Lohynska, R.; Daugaard, G.; Richard, S.; Chompret, A.; Bonaiti-Pellie, C.; Heidenreich, A.; Albers, P.; Olah, E.; Geczi, L.; Bodrogi, I.; Ormiston, W.J.; Daly, P.A.; Guilford, P.; Fossa, S.D.; Heimdal, K.; Tjulandin, S.A.; Liubchenko, L.; Stoll, H.; Weber, W.; Forman, D.; Oliver, T.; Einhorn, L.; McMaster, M.; Kramer, J.; Greene, M.H.; Weber, B.L.; Nathanson, K.L.; Cortessis, V.; Easton, D.F.; Bishop, D.T.; Stratton, M.R. & Rapley, E.A. (2006). Genome-wide linkage screen for testicular germ cell tumour susceptibility loci. *Hum Mol Genet,* Vol.15, No.3, (Februar 2006), pp.443-451, ISSN 0964-6906

Crowder, R.J.; Enomoto, H.; Yang, M.; Johnson, E.M., Jr. & Milbrandt, J. (2004). Dok-6, a Novel p62 Dok family member, promotes Ret-mediated neurite outgrowth. *J Biol Chem,* Vol.279, No.40, (October 2004), pp.42072-42081, ISSN 0021-9258

Danchin, E.; Charmantier, A.; Champagne, F.A.; Mesoudi, A.; Pujol, B. & Blanchet, S. (2011). Beyond DNA: integrating inclusive inheritance into an extended theory of evolution. *Nat Rev Genet,* Vol.12, No.7, (July 2011), pp.475-486, ISSN 1471-0064

de Rooij, D.G. (2001). Proliferation and differentiation of spermatogonial stem cells. *Reproduction,* Vol.121, No.3, (March 2001), pp.347-354, ISSN 1470-1626

Di Cristofano, A.; Pesce, B.; Cordon-Cardo, C. & Pandolfi, P.P. (1998). Pten is essential for embryonic development and tumour suppression. *Nat Genet,* Vol.19, No.4, (August 1998), pp.348-355, ISSN 1061-4036

Dieckmann, K.P. & Pichlmeier, U. (2004). Clinical epidemiology of testicular germ cell tumors. *World J Urol,* Vol.22, No.1, (April 2004), pp.2-14, ISSN 0724-4983

Donehower, L.A.; Harvey, M.; Slagle, B.L.; McArthur, M.J.; Montgomery, C.A., Jr.; Butel, J.S. & Bradley, A. (1992). Mice deficient for p53 are developmentally normal but susceptible to spontaneous tumours. *Nature,* Vol.356, No.6366, (March 1992), pp.215-221, ISSN 0028-0836

Donehower, L.A.; Harvey, M.; Vogel, H.; McArthur, M.J.; Montgomery, C.A., Jr.; Park, S.H.; Thompson, T.; Ford, R.J. & Bradley, A. (1995). Effects of genetic background on tumorigenesis in p53-deficient mice. *Mol Carcinog,* Vol.14, No.1, (September 1995), pp.16-22, ISSN 0899-1987

Donovan, P.J. (1998). The germ cell—the mother of all stem cells. *Int. J. Dev. Biol.,* Vol.42, No.7, (1998), pp.1043-1050, ISSN 1696-3547

Duhl, D.M.; Stevens, M.E.; Vrieling, H.; Saxon, P.J.; Miller, M.W.; Epstein, C.J. & Barsh, G.S. (1994). Pleiotropic effects of the mouse lethal yellow (Ay) mutation explained by deletion of a maternally expressed gene and the simultaneous production of agouti fusion RNAs. *Development,* Vol.120, No.6, (June 1994), pp.1695-1708, ISSN 0950-1991

Ehrmann, I.E.; Ellis, P.S.; Mazeyrat, S.; Duthie, S.; Brockdorff, N.; Mattei, M.G.; Gavin, M.A.; Affara, N.A.; Brown, G.M.; Simpson, E.; Mitchell, M.J. & Scott, D.M. (1998). Characterization of genes encoding translation initiation factor eIF-2gamma in mouse and human: sex chromosome localization, escape from X-inactivation and evolution. *Hum Mol Genet,* Vol.7, No.11, (October 1998), pp.1725-1737, ISSN 0964-6906

Fahrioglu, U.; Murphy, M.W.; Zarkower, D. & Bardwell, V.J. (2007). mRNA expression analysis and the molecular basis of neonatal testis defects in Dmrt1 mutant mice. *Sex Dev,* Vol.1, No.1, (April 2007), pp.42-58, ISSN 1661-5433

Flanagan, J.G.; Chan, D.C. & Leder, P. (1991). Transmembrane form of the kit ligand growth factor is determined by alternative splicing and is missing in the Sld mutant. *Cell,* Vol.64, No.5, (March 1991), pp.1025-1035, ISSN 0092-8674

Fu, Y.H.; Kuhl, D.P.; Pizzuti, A.; Pieretti, M.; Sutcliffe, J.S.; Richards, S.; Verkerk, A.J.; Holden, J.J.; Fenwick, R.G., Jr.; Warren, S.T. et al. (1991). Variation of the CGG repeat at the fragile X site results in genetic instability: resolution of the Sherman paradox. *Cell,* Vol.67, No.6, (December 1991), pp.1047-1058, ISSN 0092-8674

Gilbert, D.; Rapley, E. & Shipley, J. (2011). Testicular germ cell tumours: predisposition genes and the male germ cell niche. *Nat Rev Cancer,* Vol.11, No.4, (April 2011), pp.278-288, ISSN 1474-1768

Giwercman, A. & Giwercman, Y.L. (2011). Environmental factors and testicular function. *Best Pract Res Clin Endocrinol Metab,* Vol.25, No.2, (April 2011), pp.391-402, ISSN 1532-1908

Grieco, M.; Santoro, M.; Berlingieri, M.T.; Melillo, R.M.; Donghi, R.; Bongarzone, I.; Pierotti, M.A.; Della Porta, G.; Fusco, A. & Vecchio, G. (1990). PTC is a novel rearranged form of the ret proto-oncogene and is frequently detected in vivo in human thyroid papillary carcinomas. *Cell,* Vol.60, No.4, (Februar 1990), pp.557-563, ISSN 0092-8674

Griswold, M.D. (1995). Interactions between germ cells and Sertoli cells in the testis. *Biol Reprod,* Vol.52, No.2, (Februar 1995), pp.211-216, ISSN 0006-3363

Gustavson, K.H.; Gamstorp, I. & Meurling, S. (1975). Bilateral teratoma of testis in two brothers with 47,XXY Klinefelter's syndrome. *Clin Genet,* Vol.8, No.1, (July 1975), pp.5-10, ISSN 0009-9163

Hammond, S.; Zhu, R.; Youngren, K.K.; Lam, J.; Anderson, P. & Matin, A. (2007). Chromosome X modulates incidence of testicular germ cell tumors in *Ter* mice. *Mamm Genome,* Vol.18, No.12, (December 2007), pp.832-838, ISSN 0938-8990

Hayashi, K.; Chuva de Sousa Lopes, S.M.; Kaneda, M.; Tang, F.; Hajkova, P.; Lao, K.; O'Carroll, D.; Das, P.P.; Tarakhovsky, A.; Miska, E.A. & Surani, M.A. (2008). MicroRNA biogenesis is required for mouse primordial germ cell development and spermatogenesis. *PLoS One,* Vol.3, No.3, (March 2008), pp.e1738, ISSN 1932-6203

He, X.; Ni, Y.; Wang, Y.; Romigh, T. & Eng, C. (2011). Naturally occurring germline and tumor-associated mutations within the ATP-binding motifs of PTEN lead to oxidative damage of DNA associated with decreased nuclear p53. *Hum Mol Genet,* Vol.20, No.1, (January 2011), pp.80-89, ISSN 1460-2083

Heaney, J.D.; Lam, M.Y.; Michelson, M.V. & Nadeau, J.H. (2008). Loss of the transmembrane but not the soluble kit ligand isoform increases testicular germ cell tumor susceptibility in mice. *Cancer Res,* Vol.68, No.13, (July 2008), pp.5193-5197, ISSN 1538-7445

Heaney, J.D.; Michelson, M.V.; Youngren, K.K.; Lam, M.Y. & Nadeau, J.H. (2009). Deletion of eIF2beta suppresses testicular cancer incidence and causes recessive lethality in agouti-yellow mice. *Hum Mol Genet,* Vol.18, No.8, (April 2009), pp.1395-1404, ISSN 1460-2083

Heiss, N.S.; Knight, S.W.; Vulliamy, T.J.; Klauck, S.M.; Wiemann, S.; Mason, P.J.; Poustka, A. & Dokal, I. (1998). X-linked dyskeratosis congenita is caused by mutations in a highly conserved gene with putative nucleolar functions. *Nat Genet,* Vol.19, No.1, (May 1998), pp.32-38, ISSN 1061-4036

Hess, R.A.; Cooke, P.S.; Hofmann, M.C. & Murphy, K.M. (2006). Mechanistic insights into the regulation of the spermatogonial stem cell niche. *Cell Cycle,* Vol.5, No.11, (June 2006), pp.1164-1170, ISSN 1551-4005

Huang, E.J.; Nocka, K.H.; Buck, J. & Besmer, P. (1992). Differential expression and processing of two cell associated forms of the kit-ligand: KL-1 and KL-2. *Mol Biol Cell,* Vol.3, No.3, (March 1992), pp.349-362, ISSN 1059-1524

Hutter, A.M., Jr.; Lynch, J.L. & Schnider, B.I. (1967). Malignant testicular tumors in brothers. *JAMA,* Vol.199, No.13, (March 1967), pp.155-156, ISSN 0098-7484

Ishii, T.; Kohu, K.; Yamada, S.; Ishidoya, S.; Kanto, S.; Fuji, H.; Moriya, T.; Satake, M. & Arai, Y. (2007). Up-regulation of DNA-methyltransferase 3A expression is associated with hypomethylation of intron 25 in human testicular germ cell tumors. *Tohoku J Exp Med,* Vol.212, No.2, (June 2007), pp.177-190, ISSN 0040-8727

Jacks, T.; Remington, L.; Williams, B.O.; Schmitt, E.M.; Halachmi, S.; Bronson, R.T. & Weinberg, R.A. (1994). Tumor spectrum analysis in p53-mutant mice. *Curr Biol,* Vol.4, No.1, (January 1994), pp.1-7, ISSN 0960-9822

Jady, B.E.; Bertrand, E. & Kiss, T. (2004). Human telomerase RNA and box H/ACA scaRNAs share a common Cajal body-specific localization signal. *J Cell Biol,* Vol.164, No.5, (March 2004), pp.647-652, ISSN 0021-9525

Jin, P.; Zarnescu, D.C.; Ceman, S.; Nakamoto, M.; Mowrey, J.; Jongens, T.A.; Nelson, D.L.; Moses, K. & Warren, S.T. (2004). Biochemical and genetic interaction between the fragile X mental retardation protein and the microRNA pathway. *Nat Neurosci,* Vol.7, No.2, (Februar 2004), pp.113-117, ISSN 1097-6256

Jordan, S.A.; Speed, R.M.; Bernex, F. & Jackson, I.J. (1999). Deficiency of Trp53 rescues the male fertility defects of Kit(W-v) mice but has no effect on the survival of melanocytes and mast cells. *Dev Biol,* Vol.215, No.1, (November 1999), pp.78-90, ISSN 0012-1606

Kalfa, N.; Paris, F.; Soyer-Gobillard, M.O.; Daures, J.P. & Sultan, C. (2011). Prevalence of hypospadias in grandsons of women exposed to diethylstilbestrol during pregnancy: a multigenerational national cohort study. *Fertil Steril,* Vol.95, No.8, (June 2011), pp.2574-2577, ISSN 1556-5653

Kanetsky, P.A.; Mitra, N.; Vardhanabhuti, S.; Li, M.; Vaughn, D.J.; Letrero, R.; Ciosek, S.L.; Doody, D.R.; Smith, L.M.; Weaver, J.; Albano, A.; Chen, C.; Starr, J.R.; Rader, D.J.; Godwin, A.K.; Reilly, M.P.; Hakonarson, H.; Schwartz, S.M. & Nathanson, K.L. (2009). Common variation in KITLG and at 5q31.3 predisposes to testicular germ cell cancer. *Nat Genet,* Vol.41, No.7, (July 2009), pp.811-815, ISSN 1546-1718

Kanetsky, P.A.; Mitra, N.; Vardhanabhuti, S.; Vaughn, D.J.; Li, M.; Ciosek, S.L.; Letrero, R.; D'Andrea, K.; Vaddi, M.; Doody, D.R.; Weaver, J.; Chen, C.; Starr, J.R.; Hakonarson, H.; Rader, D.J.; Godwin, A.K.; Reilly, M.P.; Schwartz, S.M. & Nathanson, K.L.

(2011). A second independent locus within DMRT1 is associated with testicular germ cell tumor susceptibility. *Hum Mol Genet,* Vol.20, No.15, (August 2011), pp.3109-3117, ISSN 1460-2083

Karl, J. & Capel, B. (1998). Sertoli cells of the mouse testis originate from the coelomic epithelium. *Dev Biol,* Vol.203, No.2, (November 1998), pp.323-333, ISSN 0012-1606

Kedde, M.; Strasser, M.J.; Boldajipour, B.; Oude Vrielink, J.A.; Slanchev, K.; le Sage, C.; Nagel, R.; Voorhoeve, P.M.; van Duijse, J.; Orom, U.A.; Lund, A.H.; Perrakis, A.; Raz, E. & Agami, R. (2007). RNA-binding protein Dnd1 inhibits microRNA access to target mRNA. *Cell,* Vol.131, No.7, (December 2007), pp.1273-1286, ISSN 0092-8674

Kimura, T.; Suzuki, A.; Fujita, Y.; Yomogida, K.; Lomeli, H.; Asada, N.; Ikeuchi, M.; Nagy, A.; Mak, T.W. & Nakano, T. (2003). Conditional loss of PTEN leads to testicular teratoma and enhances embryonic germ cell production. *Development,* Vol.130, No.8, (April 2003), pp.1691-1700, ISSN 0950-1991

Kissel, H.; Timokhina, I.; Hardy, M.P.; Rothschild, G.; Tajima, Y.; Soares, V.; Angeles, M.; Whitlow, S.R.; Manova, K. & Besmer, P. (2000). Point mutation in kit receptor tyrosine kinase reveals essential roles for kit signaling in spermatogenesis and oogenesis without affecting other kit responses. *EMBO J,* Vol.19, No.6, (March 2000), pp.1312-1326, ISSN 0261-4189

Koubova, J.; Menke, D.B.; Zhou, Q.; Capel, B.; Griswold, M.D. & Page, D.C. (2006). Retinoic acid regulates sex-specific timing of meiotic initiation in mice. *Proc Natl Acad Sci U S A,* Vol.103, No.8, (Februar 2006), pp.2474-2479, ISSN 0027-8424

Kouprina, N.; Mullokandov, M.; Rogozin, I.B.; Collins, N.K.; Solomon, G.; Otstot, J.; Risinger, J.I.; Koonin, E.V.; Barrett, J.C. & Larionov, V. (2004). The SPANX gene family of cancer/testis-specific antigens: rapid evolution and amplification in African great apes and hominids. *Proc Natl Acad Sci U S A,* Vol.101, No.9, (March 2004), pp.3077-3082, ISSN 0027-8424

Krentz, A.D.; Murphy, M.W.; Kim, S.; Cook, M.S.; Capel, B.; Zhu, R.; Matin, A.; Sarver, A.L.; Parker, K.L.; Griswold, M.D.; Looijenga, L.H.; Bardwell, V.J. & Zarkower, D. (2009). The DM domain protein DMRT1 is a dose-sensitive regulator of fetal germ cell proliferation and pluripotency. *Proc Natl Acad Sci U S A,* Vol.106, No.52, (December 2009), pp.22323-22328, ISSN 1091-6490

Krishna, S.; Low, I.C. & Pervaiz, S. (2011). Regulation of mitochondrial metabolism: yet another facet in the biology of the oncoprotein Bcl-2. *Biochem J,* Vol.435, No.3, (May 2011), pp.545-551, ISSN 1470-8728

Lam, M.Y.; Youngren, K.K. & Nadeau, J.H. (2004). Enhancers and suppressors of testicular cancer susceptibility in single- and double-mutant mice. *Genetics,* Vol.166, No.2, (Februar 2004), pp.925-933, ISSN 0016-6731

Lam, M.Y.; Heaney, J.D.; Youngren, K.K.; Kawasoe, J.H. & Nadeau, J.H. (2007). Trans-generational epistasis between Dnd1Ter and other modifier genes controls susceptibility to testicular germ cell tumors. *Hum Mol Genet,* Vol.16, No.18, (September 2007), pp.2233-2240, ISSN 0964-6906

Lambrot, R.; Coffigny, H.; Pairault, C.; Lecureuil, C.; Frydman, R.; Habert, R. & Rouiller-Fabre, V. (2007). High radiosensitivity of germ cells in human male fetus. *J Clin Endocrinol Metab,* Vol.92, No.7, (July 2007), pp.2632-2639, ISSN 0021-972X

Lau, M.T.; Klausen, C. & Leung, P.C. (2011). E-cadherin inhibits tumor cell growth by suppressing PI3K/Akt signaling via beta-catenin-Egr1-mediated PTEN expression. *Oncogene,* Vol.30, No.24, (June 2011), pp.2753-2766, ISSN 1476-5594

Lau, Y.F. (1999). Gonadoblastoma, testicular and prostate cancers, and the TSPY gene. *Am J Hum Genet,* Vol.64, No.4, (April 1999), pp.921-927, ISSN 0002-9297

LeBron, C.; Pal, P.; Brait, M.; Dasgupta, S.; Guerrero-Preston, R.; Looijenga, L.H.; Kowalski, J.; Netto, G. & Hoque, M.O. (2011). Genome-wide analysis of genetic alterations in testicular primary seminoma using high resolution single nucleotide polymorphism arrays. *Genomics,* Vol.97, No.6, (June 2011), pp.341-349, ISSN 1089-8646

Lee, H.W.; Blasco, M.A.; Gottlieb, G.J.; Horner, J.W., 2nd; Greider, C.W. & DePinho, R.A. (1998). Essential role of mouse telomerase in highly proliferative organs. *Nature,* Vol.392, No.6676, (April 1998), pp.569-574, ISSN 0028-0836

Leeksma, O.C.; Van Achterberg, T.A.; Tsumura, Y.; Toshima, J.; Eldering, E.; Kroes, W.G.; Mellink, C.; Spaargaren, M.; Mizuno, K.; Pannekoek, H. & de Vries, C.J. (2002). Human sprouty 4, a new ras antagonist on 5q31, interacts with the dual specificity kinase TESK1. *Eur J Biochem,* Vol.269, No.10, (May 2002), pp.2546-2556, ISSN 0014-2956

Li, H.; MacLean, G.; Cameron, D.; Clagett-Dame, M. & Petkovich, M. (2009). Cyp26b1 expression in murine Sertoli cells is required to maintain male germ cells in an undifferentiated state during embryogenesis. *PLoS One,* Vol.4, No.10, (October 2009), pp.e7501, ISSN 1932-6203

Lin, T.; Chao, C.; Saito, S.; Mazur, S.J.; Murphy, M.E.; Appella, E. & Xu, Y. (2005). p53 induces differentiation of mouse embryonic stem cells by suppressing Nanog expression. *Nat Cell Biol,* Vol.7, No.2, (Februar 2005), pp.165-171, ISSN 1465-7392

Liu, D.; Ou, L.; Clemenson, G.D., Jr.; Chao, C.; Lutske, M.E.; Zambetti, G.P.; Gage, F.H. & Xu, Y. (2010). Puma is required for p53-induced depletion of adult stem cells. *Nat Cell Biol,* Vol.12, No.10, (October 2010), pp.993-998, ISSN 1476-4679

Liu, Z.; Luyten, I.; Bottomley, M.J.; Messias, A.C.; Houngninou-Molango, S.; Sprangers, R.; Zanier, K.; Kramer, A. & Sattler, M. (2001). Structural basis for recognition of the intron branch site RNA by splicing factor 1. *Science,* Vol.294, No.5544, (November 2001), pp.1098-1102, ISSN 0036-8075

Lobo, G.P.; Waite, K.A.; Planchon, S.M.; Romigh, T.; Nassif, N.T. & Eng, C. (2009). Germline and somatic cancer-associated mutations in the ATP-binding motifs of PTEN influence its subcellular localization and tumor suppressive function. *Hum Mol Genet,* Vol.18, No.15, (August 2009), pp.2851-2862, ISSN 1460-2083

Looijenga, L.H.; de Leeuw, H.; van Oorschot, M.; van Gurp, R.J.; Stoop, H.; Gillis, A.J.; de Gouveia Brazao, C.A.; Weber, R.F.; Kirkels, W.J.; van Dijk, T.; von Lindern, M.; Valk, P.; Lajos, G.; Olah, E.; Nesland, J.M.; Fossa, S.D. & Oosterhuis, J.W. (2003). Stem cell factor receptor (c-KIT) codon 816 mutations predict development of bilateral testicular germ-cell tumors. *Cancer Res,* Vol.63, No.22, (November 2003), pp.7674-7678, ISSN 0008-5472

MacLean, G.; Li, H.; Metzger, D.; Chambon, P. & Petkovich, M. (2007). Apoptotic extinction of germ cells in testes of Cyp26b1 knockout mice. *Endocrinology,* Vol.148, No.10, (October 2007), pp.4560-4567, ISSN 0013-7227

Mahmoudi, S.; Henriksson, S.; Corcoran, M.; Mendez-Vidal, C.; Wiman, K.G. & Farnebo, M. (2009). Wrap53, a natural p53 antisense transcript required for p53 induction upon DNA damage. *Mol Cell,* Vol.33, No.4, (Februar 2009), pp.462-471, ISSN 1097-4164

Malkin, D.; Li, F.P.; Strong, L.C.; Fraumeni, J.F.Jr.; Nelson, C.E.; Kim, D.H.; Kassel, J.; Gryka, M.A.; Bischoff, F.Z.; Tainsky, M.A. & Friend, S.H. (1990). Germ line p53 mutations in a familial syndrome of breast cancer, sarcomas, and other neoplasms. *Science,* Vol.250, No.4985, (September 1990), pp.1233-1238, ISSN 0036-8075

Manova, K.; Nocka, K.; Besmer, P. & Bachvarova, R.F. (1990). Gonadal expression of c-kit encoded at the W locus of the mouse. *Development,* Vol.110, No.4, (December 1990), pp.1057-1069, ISSN 0950-1991

Marrone, A.; Walne, A.; Tamary, H.; Masunari, Y.; Kirwan, M.; Beswick, R.; Vulliamy, T. & Dokal, I. (2007). Telomerase reverse-transcriptase homozygous mutations in autosomal recessive dyskeratosis congenita and Hoyeraal-Hreidarsson syndrome. *Blood,* Vol.110, No.13, (December 2007), pp.4198-4205, ISSN 0006-4971

Matin, A.; Collin, G.B.; Asada, Y.; Varnum, D.; Martone, D.L. & Nadeau, J.H. (1998). Simple sequence length polymorphisms (SSLPs) that distinguish MOLF/Ei and 129/Sv inbred strains of laboratory mice. *Mamm Genome,* Vol.9, No.8, (August 1998), pp.668-670, ISSN 0938-8990

Matin, A.; Collin, G.B.; Asada, Y.; Varnum, D. & Nadeau, J.H. (1999). Susceptibility to testicular germ-cell tumours in a 129.MOLF-Chr 19 chromosome substitution strain. *Nat Genet,* Vol.23, No.2, (October 1999), pp.237-240, ISSN 1061-4036

Matson, C.K.; Murphy, M.W.; Griswold, M.D.; Yoshida, S.; Bardwell, V.J. & Zarkower, D. (2010). The mammalian doublesex homolog DMRT1 is a transcriptional gatekeeper that controls the mitosis versus meiosis decision in male germ cells. *Dev Cell,* Vol.19, No.4, (October 2010), pp.612-624, ISSN 1878-1551

Matsui, Y.; Zsebo, K.M. & Hogan, B.L. (1990). Embryonic expression of a haematopoietic growth factor encoded by the Sl locus and the ligand for c-kit. *Nature,* Vol.347, No.6294, (October 1990), pp.667-669, ISSN 0028-0836

Mauduit, C.; Hamamah, S. & Benahmed, M. (1999). Stem cell factor/c-kit system in spermatogenesis. *Hum Reprod Update,* Vol.5, No.5, (October 1999), pp.535-545, ISSN 1355-4786

McConkie-Rosell, A.; Lachiewicz, A.M.; Spiridigliozzi, G.A.; Tarleton, J.; Schoenwald, S.; Phelan, M.C.; Goonewardena, P.; Ding, X. & Brown, W.T. (1993). Evidence that methylation of the FMR-I locus is responsible for variable phenotypic expression of the fragile X syndrome. *Am J Hum Genet,* Vol.53, No.4, (October 1993), pp.800-809, ISSN 0002-9297

McCoshen, J.A. & McCallion, D.J. (1975). A study of the primordial germ cells during their migratory phase in Steel mutant mice. *Experientia,* Vol.31, No.5, (May 1975), pp.589-590, ISSN 0014-4754

McGlynn, K.A.; Devesa, S.S.; Graubard, B.I. & Castle, P.E. (2005). Increasing incidence of testicular germ cell tumors among black men in the United States. *J Clin Oncol,* Vol.23, No.24, (August 2005), pp.5757-5761, ISSN 0732-183X

Michalak, E.; Villunger, A.; Erlacher, M. & Strasser, A. (2005). Death squads enlisted by the tumour suppressor p53. *Biochem Biophys Res Commun,* Vol.331, No.3, (June 2005), pp.786-798, ISSN 0006-291X

Michaud, E.J.; Bultman, S.J.; Klebig, M.L.; van Vugt, M.J.; Stubbs, L.J.; Russell, L.B. & Woychik, R.P. (1994). A molecular model for the genetic and phenotypic characteristics of the mouse lethal yellow (Ay) mutation. *Proc Natl Acad Sci U S A,* Vol.91, No.7, (March 1994), pp.2562-2566, ISSN 0027-8424

Mieno, M.; Udono, H.; Ikegami, S.; Tada, N.; Shiku, H. & Nakayama, E. (1989). Blocking of cytotoxic T-cell function of MOLF/Ei mice by anti-Ly 35.1 monoclonal antibody. *Immunology,* Vol.68, No.3, (November 1989), pp.431-433, ISSN 0019-2805

Minami, K.; Chano, T.; Kawakami, T.; Ushida, H.; Kushima, R.; Okabe, H.; Okada, Y. & Okamoto, K. (2010). DNMT3L is a novel marker and is essential for the growth of human embryonal carcinoma. *Clin Cancer Res,* Vol.16, No.10, (May 2010), pp.2751-2759, ISSN 1078-0432

Mithraprabhu, S. & Loveland, K.L. (2009). Control of KIT signalling in male germ cells: what can we learn from other systems? *Reproduction,* Vol.138, No.5, (November 2009), pp.743-757, ISSN 1741-7899

Molyneaux, K.A.; Stallock, J.; Schaible, K. & Wylie, C. (2001). Time-lapse analysis of living mouse germ cell migration. *Dev Biol,* Vol.240, No.2, (December 2001), pp.488-498, ISSN 0012-1606

Moore, F.L.; Jaruzelska, J.; Fox, M.S.; Urano, J.; Firpo, M.T.; Turek, P.J.; Dorfman, D.M. & Pera, R.A. (2003). Human Pumilio-2 is expressed in embryonic stem cells and germ cells and interacts with DAZ (Deleted in AZoospermia) and DAZ-like proteins. *Proc Natl Acad Sci U S A,* Vol.100, No.2, (January 2003), pp.538-543, ISSN 0027-8424

Muller, A.J.; Teresky, A.K. & Levine, A.J. (2000). A male germ cell tumor-susceptibility-determining locus, pgct1, identified on murine chromosome 13. *Proc Natl Acad Sci U S A,* Vol.97, No.15, (July 2000), pp.8421-8426, ISSN 0027-8424

Murphy, M.W.; Sarver, A.L.; Rice, D.; Hatzi, K.; Ye, K.; Melnick, A.; Heckert, L.L.; Zarkower, D. & Bardwell, V.J. (2010). Genome-wide analysis of DNA binding and transcriptional regulation by the mammalian Doublesex homolog DMRT1 in the juvenile testis. *Proc Natl Acad Sci U S A,* Vol.107, No.30, (July 2010), pp.13360-13365, ISSN 1091-6490

Murty, V.V.; Houldsworth, J.; Baldwin, S.; Reuter, V.; Hunziker, W.; Besmer, P.; Bosl, G. & Chaganti, R.S. (1992). Allelic deletions in the long arm of chromosome 12 identify sites of candidate tumor suppressor genes in male germ cell tumors. *Proc Natl Acad Sci U S A,* Vol.89, No.22, (November 1992), pp.11006-11010, ISSN 0027-8424

Murty, V.V.; Bosl, G.J.; Houldsworth, J.; Meyers, M.; Mukherjee, A.B.; Reuter, V. & Chaganti, R.S. (1994). Allelic loss and somatic differentiation in human male germ cell tumors. *Oncogene,* Vol.9, No.8, (August 1994), pp.2245-2251, ISSN 0950-9232

Myers, M.P.; Stolarov, J.P.; Eng, C.; Li, J.; Wang, S.I.; Wigler, M.H.; Parsons, R. & Tonks, N.K. (1997). P-TEN, the tumor suppressor from human chromosome 10q23, is a dual-specificity phosphatase. *Proc Natl Acad Sci U S A,* Vol.94, No.17, (August 1997), pp.9052-9057, ISSN 0027-8424

Nagano, R.; Tabata, S.; Nakanishi, Y.; Ohsako, S.; Kurohmaru, M. & Hayashi, Y. (2000). Reproliferation and relocation of mouse male germ cells (gonocytes) during prespermatogenesis. *Anat Rec,* Vol.258, No.2, (Februar 2000), pp.210-220, ISSN 0003-276X

Nathanson, K.L.; Kanetsky, P.A.; Hawes, R.; Vaughn, D.J.; Letrero, R.; Tucker, K.; Friedlander, M.; Phillips, K.A.; Hogg, D.; Jewett, M.A.; Lohynska, R.; Daugaard, G.;

Richard, S.; Chompret, A.; Bonaiti-Pellie, C.; Heidenreich, A. et al. (2005). The Y deletion gr/gr and susceptibility to testicular germ cell tumor. *Am J Hum Genet,* Vol.77, No.6, (December 2005), pp.1034-1043, ISSN 0002-9297

Nelson, K.M. & Weiss, G.J. (2008). MicroRNAs and cancer: past, present, and potential future. *Mol Cancer Ther,* Vol.7, No.12, (December 2008), pp.3655-3660, ISSN 1535-7163

Nelson, V.R. & Nadeau J.H. (2010) Transgenerational genetic effects. *Epigenomics,* Vol.2, No.6, pp.797-806, ISSN 1750-1911

Nocka, K.; Buck, J.; Levi, E. & Besmer, P. (1990). Candidate ligand for the c-kit transmembrane kinase receptor: KL, a fibroblast derived growth factor stimulates mast cells and erythroid progenitors. *EMBO J,* Vol.9, No.10, (October 1990), pp.3287-3294, ISSN 0261-4189

Noguchi, T. & Noguchi, M. (1985). A recessive mutation (ter) causing germ cell deficiency and a high incidence of congenital testicular teratomas in 129/Sv-ter mice. *J Natl Cancer Inst,* Vol.75, No.2, (August 1985), pp.385-392, ISSN 0027-8874

Parker, R. & Sheth, U. (2007). P bodies and the control of mRNA translation and degradation. *Mol Cell,* Vol.25, No.5, (March 2007), pp.635-646, ISSN 1097-2765

Patriotis, C.; Makris, A.; Chernoff, J. & Tsichlis, P.N. (1994). Tpl-2 acts in concert with Ras and Raf-1 to activate mitogen-activated protein kinase. *Proc Natl Acad Sci U S A,* Vol.91, No.21, (October 1994), pp.9755-9759, ISSN 0027-8424

Peltomaki, P.; Halme, A. & de la Chapelle, A. (1990). Human testicular cancer. Changes in autosomal dosage. *Cancer Genet Cytogenet,* Vol.48, No.1, (August 1990), pp.1-12, ISSN 0165-4608

Peng, H.Q.; Bailey, D.; Bronson, D.; Goss, P.E. & Hogg, D. (1995). Loss of heterozygosity of tumor suppressor genes in testis cancer. *Cancer Res,* Vol.55, No.13, (July 1995), pp.2871-2875, ISSN 0008-5472

Pesce, M.; Farrace, M.G.; Piacentini, M.; Dolci, S. & De Felici, M. (1993). Stem cell factor and leukemia inhibitory factor promote primordial germ cell survival by suppressing programmed cell death (apoptosis). *Development,* Vol.118, No.4, (August 1993), pp.1089-1094, ISSN 0950-1991

Rapley, E.A.; Crockford, G.P.; Teare, D.; Biggs, P.; Seal, S.; Barfoot, R.; Edwards, S.; Hamoudi, R.; Heimdal, K.; Fossa, S.D.; Tucker, K.; Donald, J.; Collins, F.; Friedlander, M.; Hogg, D.; Goss, P.; Heidenreich, A.; Olah, E.; Geczi, L.; Bodrogi, I.; Ormiston, W.J.; Daly, P.A.; Oosterhuis, J.W.; Gillis, A.J.; Looijenga, L.H.; Guilford, P.; Fossa, S.D.; Heimdal, K.; Tjulandin, S.A.; Liubchenko, L.; Stoll, H.; Weber, W.; Rudd, M.; Huddart, R.; Crockford, G.P.; Forman, D.; Oliver, D.T.; Einhorn, L.; Weber, B.L.; Kramer, J.; McMaster, M.; Greene, M.H.; Pike, M.; Cortessis, V.; Chen, C.; Schwartz, S.M.; Bishop, D.T.; Easton, D.F.; Stratton, M.R. & Rapley, E.A. (2000). Localization to Xq27 of a susceptibility gene for testicular germ-cell tumours. *Nat Genet,* Vol.24, No.2, (Februar 2000), pp.197-200, ISSN 1061-4036

Rapley, E.A.; Turnbull, C.; Al Olama, A.A.; Dermitzakis, E.T.; Linger, R.; Huddart, R.A.; Renwick, A.; Hughes, D.; Hines, S.; Seal, S.; Morrison, J.; Nsengimana, J.; Deloukas, P.; Rahman, N.; Bishop, D.T.; Easton, D.F. & Stratton, M.R. (2009). A genome-wide association study of testicular germ cell tumor. *Nat Genet,* Vol.41, No.7, (July 2009), pp.807-810, ISSN 1546-1718

Raymond, C.S.; Kettlewell, J.R.; Hirsch, B.; Bardwell, V.J. & Zarkower, D. (1999). Expression of Dmrt1 in the genital ridge of mouse and chicken embryos suggests a role in vertebrate sexual development. *Dev Biol,* Vol.215, No.2, (November 1999), pp.208-220, ISSN 0012-1606

Raymond, C.S.; Murphy, M.W.; O'Sullivan, M.G.; Bardwell, V.J. & Zarkower, D. (2000). Dmrt1, a gene related to worm and fly sexual regulators, is required for mammalian testis differentiation. *Genes Dev,* Vol.14, No.20, (October 2000), pp.2587-2595, ISSN 0890-9369

Rivers, E.N. & Hamilton, D.W. (1986). Morphologic analysis of spontaneous teratocarcinogenesis in developing testes of strain 129/Sv-ter mice. *Am J Pathol,* Vol.124, No.2, (August 1986), pp.263-280, ISSN 0002-9440

Rossi, P.; Albanesi, C.; Grimaldi, P. & Geremia, R. (1991). Expression of the mRNA for the ligand of c-kit in mouse Sertoli cells. *Biochem Biophys Res Commun,* Vol.176, No.2, (April 1991), pp.910-914, ISSN 0006-291X

Rotter, V.; Schwartz, D.; Almon, E.; Goldfinger, N.; Kapon, A.; Meshorer, A.; Donehower, L.A. & Levine, A.J. (1993). Mice with reduced levels of p53 protein exhibit the testicular giant-cell degenerative syndrome. *Proc Natl Acad Sci U S A,* Vol.90, No.19, (October 1993), pp.9075-9079, ISSN 0027-8424

Saal, L.H.; Gruvberger-Saal, S.K.; Persson, C.; Lovgren, K.; Jumppanen, M.; Staaf, J.; Jonsson, G.; Pires, M.M.; Maurer, M.; Holm, K.; Koujak, S.; Subramaniyam, S.; Vallon-Christersson, J.; Olsson, H.; Su, T.; Memeo, L.; Ludwig, T. et al. (2008). Recurrent gross mutations of the PTEN tumor suppressor gene in breast cancers with deficient DSB repair. *Nat Genet,* Vol.40, No.1, (January 2008), pp.102-107, ISSN 1546-1718

Salemi, M.; Calogero, A.E.; Castiglione, R.; Tricoli, D.; Asero, P.; Rosa, R.; Rappazzo, G. & Vicari, E. (2006). Expression of SpanX proteins in normal testes and in testicular germ cell tumours. *Int J Androl,* Vol.29, No.2, (April 2006), pp.368-373, ISSN 0105-6263

Sarre, T.F. (1989). The phosphorylation of eukaryotic initiation factor 2: a principle of translational control in mammalian cells. *Biosystems,* Vol.22, No.4, pp.311-325, ISSN 0303-2647

Sasaki, H. & Matsui, Y. (2008). Epigenetic events in mammalian germ-cell development: reprogramming and beyond. *Nat Rev Genet,* Vol.9, No.2, (Februar 2008), pp.129-140, ISSN 1471-0064

Satge, D.; Sasco, A.J.; Cure, H.; Leduc, B.; Sommelet, D. & Vekemans, M.J. (1997). An excess of testicular germ cell tumors in Down's syndrome: three case reports and a review of the literature. *Cancer,* Vol.80, No.5, (September 1997), pp.929-935, ISSN 0008-543X

Schwartz, D.; Goldfinger, N. & Rotter, V. (1993). Expression of p53 protein in spermatogenesis is confined to the tetraploid pachytene primary spermatocytes. *Oncogene,* Vol.8, No.6, (June 1993), pp.1487-1494, ISSN 0950-9232

Seydoux, G. & Braun, R.E. (2006). Pathway to totipotency: lessons from germ cells. *Cell,* Vol.127, No.5, (December 2006), pp.891-904, ISSN 0092-8674

Shen, W.H.; Balajee, A.S.; Wang, J.; Wu, H.; Eng, C.; Pandolfi, P.P. & Yin, Y. (2007). Essential role for nuclear PTEN in maintaining chromosomal integrity. *Cell,* Vol.128, No.1, (January 2007), pp.157-170, ISSN 0092-8674

Shimizu, S.; Narita, M. & Tsujimoto, Y. (1999). Bcl-2 family proteins regulate the release of apoptogenic cytochrome c by the mitochondrial channel VDAC. *Nature,* Vol.399, No.6735, (June 1999), pp.483-487, ISSN 0028-0836

Skakkebaek, N.E. (1972). Abnormal morphology of germ cells in two infertile men. *Acta Pathol Microbiol Scand A,* Vol.80, No.3, pp.374-378, ISSN 0365-4184

Skotheim, R.I.; Kraggerud, S.M.; Fossa, S.D.; Stenwig, A.E.; Gedde-Dahl, T., Jr.; Danielsen, H.E.; Jakobsen, K.S. & Lothe, R.A. (2001). Familial/bilateral and sporadic testicular germ cell tumors show frequent genetic changes at loci with suggestive linkage evidence. *Neoplasia,* Vol.3, No.3, (June 2001), pp.196-203, ISSN 1522-8002

Soh, L.T.; Ang, P.T. & Lim-Tan, S.K. (1992). Embryonal carcinoma arising in Turner's syndrome. *Ann Acad Med Singapore,* Vol.21, No.3, (May 1992), pp.386-389, ISSN 0304-4602

Stallock, J.; Molyneaux, K.; Schaible, K.; Knudson, C.M. & Wylie, C. (2003). The pro-apoptotic gene Bax is required for the death of ectopic primordial germ cells during their migration in the mouse embryo. *Development,* Vol.130, No.26, (December 2003), pp.6589-6597, ISSN 0950-1991

Stevens, L.C. & Little, C.C. (1954). Spontaneous Testicular Teratomas in an Inbred Strain of Mice. *Proc Natl Acad Sci U S A,* Vol.40, No.11, (November 1954), pp.1080-1087, ISSN 0027-8424

Stevens, L.C. (1967). Origin of testicular teratomas from primordial germ cells in mice. *J Natl Cancer Inst,* Vol.38, No.4, (April 1967), pp.549-552, ISSN 0027-8874

Stevens, L.C. (1973). A new inbred subline of mice (129-terSv) with a high incidence of spontaneous congenital testicular teratomas. *J Natl Cancer Inst,* Vol.50, No.1, (January 1973), pp.235-242, ISSN 0027-8874

Su, X.; Chakravarti, D.; Cho, M.S.; Liu, L.; Gi, Y.J.; Lin, Y.L.; Leung, M.L.; El-Naggar, A.; Creighton, C.J.; Suraokar, M.B.; Wistuba, I. & Flores, E.R. (2010). TAp63 suppresses metastasis through coordinate regulation of Dicer and miRNAs. *Nature,* Vol.467, No.7318, (October 2010), pp.986-990, ISSN 1476-4687

Suzuki, A. & Saga, Y. (2008). Nanos2 suppresses meiosis and promotes male germ cell differentiation. *Genes Dev,* Vol.22, No.4, (Februar 2008), pp.430-435, ISSN 0890-9369

Suzuki, K. & Matsubara, H. (2011). Recent advances in p53 research and cancer treatment. *J Biomed Biotechnol,* Vol.2011, (July 2011), pp. 978312- 978319, ISSN 1110-7251

Swerdlow, A.J.; De Stavola, B.L.; Swanwick, M.A.; Mangtani, P. & Maconochie, N.E. (1999). Risk factors for testicular cancer: a case-control study in twins. *Br J Cancer,* Vol.80, No.7, (June 1999), pp.1098-1102, ISSN 0007-0920

Tajima, Y.; Sakamaki, K.; Watanabe, D.; Koshimizu, U.; Matsuzawa, T. & Nishimune, Y. (1991). Steel-Dickie (Sld) mutation affects both maintenance and differentiation of testicular germ cells in mice. *J Reprod Fertil,* Vol.91, No.2, (March 1991), pp.441-449, ISSN 0022-4251

Tang, Y. & Eng, C. (2006). p53 down-regulates phosphatase and tensin homologue deleted on chromosome 10 protein stability partially through caspase-mediated degradation in cells with proteasome dysfunction. *Cancer Res,* Vol.66, No.12, (June 2006), pp.6139-6148, ISSN 0008-5472

Tokuzawa, Y.; Kaiho, E.; Maruyama, M.; Takahashi, K.; Mitsui, K.; Maeda, M.; Niwa, H. & Yamanaka, S. (2003). Fbx15 is a novel target of Oct3/4 but is dispensable for embryonic stem cell self-renewal and mouse development. *Mol Cell Biol,* Vol.23, No.8, (April 2003), pp.2699-2708, ISSN 0270-7306

Tsuda, M.; Sasaoka, Y.; Kiso, M.; Abe, K.; Haraguchi, S.; Kobayashi, S. & Saga, Y. (2003). Conserved role of nanos proteins in germ cell development. *Science,* Vol.301, No.5637, (August 2003), pp.1239-1241, ISSN 1095-9203

Turnbull, C.; Rapley, E.A.; Seal, S.; Pernet, D.; Renwick, A.; Hughes, D.; Ricketts, M.; Linger, R.; Nsengimana, J.; Deloukas, P.; Huddart, R.A.; Bishop, D.T.; Easton, D.F.; Stratton, M.R. & Rahman, N. (2010). Variants near DMRT1, TERT and ATF7IP are associated with testicular germ cell cancer. *Nat Genet,* Vol.42, No.7, (July 2010), pp.604-607, ISSN 1546-1718

Ushida, H.; Kawakami, T.; Minami, K.; Chano, T.; Okabe, H.; Okada, Y. & Okamoto, K. (2011). Methylation profile of DNA repetitive elements in human testicular germ cell tumor. *Mol Carcinog,* (August 2011), ISSN 1098-2744

Venteicher, A.S.; Abreu, E.B.; Meng, Z.; McCann, K.E.; Terns, R.M.; Veenstra, T.D.; Terns, M.P. & Artandi, S.E. (2009). A human telomerase holoenzyme protein required for Cajal body localization and telomere synthesis. *Science,* Vol.323, No.5914, (January 2009), pp.644-648, ISSN 1095-9203

Vulliamy, T.; Marrone, A.; Goldman, F.; Dearlove, A.; Bessler, M.; Mason, P.J. & Dokal, I. (2001). The RNA component of telomerase is mutated in autosomal dominant dyskeratosis congenita. *Nature,* Vol.413, No.6854, (September 2001), pp.432-435, ISSN 0028-0836

Weaver, B.A.; Silk, A.D.; Montagna, C.; Verdier-Pinard, P. & Cleveland, D.W. (2007). Aneuploidy acts both oncogenically and as a tumor suppressor. *Cancer Cell,* Vol.11, No.1, (January 2007), pp.25-36, ISSN 1535-6108

Weidinger, G.; Stebler, J.; Slanchev, K.; Dumstrei, K.; Wise, C.; Lovell-Badge, R.; Thisse, C.; Thisse, B. & Raz, E. (2003). dead end, a novel vertebrate germ plasm component, is required for zebrafish primordial germ cell migration and survival. *Curr Biol,* Vol.13, No.16, (August 2003), pp.1429-1434, ISSN 0960-9822

Wendel, H.G.; De Stanchina, E.; Fridman, J.S.; Malina, A.; Ray, S.; Kogan, S.; Cordon-Cardo, C.; Pelletier, J. & Lowe, S.W. (2004). Survival signalling by Akt and eIF4E in oncogenesis and cancer therapy. *Nature,* Vol.428, No.6980, (March 2004), pp.332-337, ISSN 1476-4687

Westbrook, V.A.; Schoppee, P.D.; Diekman, A.B.; Klotz, K.L.; Allietta, M.; Hogan, K.T.; Slingluff, C.L.; Patterson, J.W.; Frierson, H.F.; Irvin, W.P., Jr.; Flickinger, C.J.; Coppola, M.A. & Herr, J.C. (2004). Genomic organization, incidence, and localization of the SPAN-x family of cancer-testis antigens in melanoma tumors and cell lines. *Clin Cancer Res,* Vol.10, No.1 Pt 1, (January 2004), pp.101-112, ISSN 1078-0432

Xu, Y. (2003). Regulation of p53 responses by post-translational modifications. *Cell Death Differ,* Vol.10, No.4, (April 2003), pp.400-403, ISSN 1350-9047

Yanagiya, A.; Delbes, G.; Svitkin, Y.V.; Robaire, B. & Sonenberg, N. (2010). The poly(A)-binding protein partner Paip2a controls translation during late spermiogenesis in mice. *J Clin Invest,* Vol.120, No.9, (September 2010), pp.3389-3400, ISSN 1558-8238

Yoshinaga, K.; Nishikawa, S.; Ogawa, M.; Hayashi, S.; Kunisada, T. & Fujimoto, T. (1991). Role of c-kit in mouse spermatogenesis: identification of spermatogonia as a specific site of c-kit expression and function. *Development,* Vol.113, No.2, (October 1991), pp.689-699, ISSN 0950-1991

Youngren, K.K.; Nadeau, J.H. & Matin, A. (2003). Testicular cancer susceptibility in the 129.MOLF-Chr19 mouse strain: additive effects, gene interactions and epigenetic modifications. *Hum Mol Genet,* Vol.12, No.4, (Februar 2003), pp.389-398, ISSN 0964-6906

Youngren, K.K.; Coveney, D.; Peng, X.; Bhattacharya, C.; Schmidt, L.S.; Nickerson, M.L.; Lamb, B.T.; Deng, J.M.; Behringer, R.R.; Capel, B.; Rubin, E.M.; Nadeau, J.H. & Matin, A. (2005). The Ter mutation in the dead end gene causes germ cell loss and testicular germ cell tumours. *Nature,* Vol.435, No.7040, (May 2005), pp.360-364, ISSN 1476-4687

Zhong, F.; Savage, S.A.; Shkreli, M.; Giri, N.; Jessop, L.; Myers, T.; Chen, R.; Alter, B.P. & Artandi, S.E. (2011). Disruption of telomerase trafficking by TCAB1 mutation causes dyskeratosis congenita. *Genes Dev,* Vol.25, No.1, (January 2011), pp.11-16, ISSN 1549-5477

Zhu, R.; Ji, Y.; Xiao, L. & Matin, A. (2007). Testicular germ cell tumor susceptibility genes from the consomic 129.MOLF-Chr19 mouse strain. *Mamm Genome,* Vol.18, No.8, (August 2007), pp.584-595, ISSN 0938-8990

Zhu, R.; Heaney, J.; Nadeau, J.H.; Ali, S. & Matin, A. (2010). Deficiency of splicing factor 1 suppresses the occurrence of testicular germ cell tumors. *Cancer Res,* Vol.70, No.18, (September 2010), pp.7264-7272, ISSN 1538-7445

Zhu, R.; Iacovino, M.; Mahen, E.; Kyba, M. & Matin, A. (2011). Transcripts that associate with the RNA binding protein, DEAD-END (DND1), in embryonic stem (ES) cells. *BMC Mol Biol,* Vol.12, No.1, (August 2011), pp.37, ISSN 1471-2199

Zhu, W.G. & Otterson, G.A. (2003). The interaction of histone deacetylase inhibitors and DNA methyltransferase inhibitors in the treatment of human cancer cells. *Curr Med Chem Anticancer Agents,* Vol.3, No.3, (May 2003), pp.187-199, ISSN 1568-0118

6

Epigenetic Modifications in Testicular Germ Cell Tumors

Christopher J. Payne
Human Molecular Genetics Program
Children's Memorial Research Center
Department of Pediatrics
Northwestern University Feinberg School of Medicine
USA

1. Introduction

Over the past decade, accumulating evidence has implicated the phenomenon of epigenetic dysregulation in a variety of cancers (Biermann and Steger, 2007). Defined as the heritable changes in gene function that are not attributable to changes in DNA sequence, epigenetics involve biochemical modifications to DNA regulatory elements as well as to the tail regions of histone proteins (Maekawa and Watanabe, 2007). Lysine and arginine residues may be acetylated and methylated, with their effect being to activate or repress gene expression in the vicinity of that specific histone modification. Promoter regions of DNA are modified through the methylation of cytosine in CpG dinucleotides, resulting in the downregulation of those genes. Recent data suggest that these epigenetic modifications play a role in the development and progression of testicular germ cell tumors (TGCTs). This chapter will focus predominantly on adult TGCTs, along with their precursor *carcinoma in situ* (CIS), and will largely exclude the distinctive pediatric/prepubertal TGCTs. Many excellent reviews describing the classification of adult TGCTs exist (see Bahrami et al., 2007), and their content will not be duplicated here. Suffice it to say that the two main categories of TGCTs will be addressed in this chapter: the relatively undifferentiated seminomas, and the more differentiated non-seminomas (ranging from the less differentiated embryonal carcinomas to the highly differentiated yolk sac tumors, teratomas, and choriocarcinomas). Examination of histone modifications, histone modifying enzymes, genes exhibiting promoter DNA hypermethylation, and DNA methyltransferases in the context of CIS, seminomas, and non-seminomas should increase our understanding of TGCT biology and potentially generate new clinical applications.

2. Histone modifications and modifying enzymes

Histone modifications greatly influence the transcription status of nearby genes in a highly specific manner. Lysine and arginine residues on the tails of histones H3 and H4 may be methylated to generate signatures that associate with active chromatin, such as the trimethylation of H3 lysine 4 (H3K4me3), or with repressed chromatin, such as the dimethylation and trimethylation of histone H3 lysine 9 (H3K9me2 and H3K9me3). Histones may also be acetylated and deacetylated through histone acetyltransferases and histone deacetylases (HDACs), which correspond to active and repressed chromatin, respectively. Histone modifying enzymes that transfer methyl groups to target residues include EZH2, SUV39H1/2, and G9a, while enzymes that remove methyl groups include JMJD3 and UTX.

2.1 H3K9 methylation

Dimethylation and trimethylation of histone H3 lysine 9 (H3K9me2 and H3K9me3) are associated with transcriptional repression. These marks are established by the histone methyltransferases SUV39H1/2 and G9a, which are critical to establish and maintain regions of heterochromatin (Peters et al., 2001; Tachibana et al., 2007). When global H3K9 methyl marks were examined in human CIS, Almstrup and colleagues found their presence to be very weak, revealing patterns similar to those in 20-40 week old normal fetal gonocytes (Almstrup et al., 2010). Interestingly, these marks were absent from the undifferentiated components of adult non-seminomatous embryonal carcinomas, but strongly detected in the undifferentiated seminomas (Almstrup et al., 2010). Godmann et al. reported the abundance of H3K9 methyl marks in both non-seminomas and seminomas, though they did not specify which nonseminomatous TGCTs they examined, nor their extent of differentiation (Godmann et al., 2009). In normal juvenile and adult mouse spermatogonia, the H3K9me2 mark is notably absent from the undifferentiated cells that exhibit stem cell activity; its presence coincides with the lineage commitment to differentiation (Payne and Braun, 2006). H3K9me3, meanwhile, exhibits a distinct perinuclear distribution in the undifferentiated germ cells that shifts and broadens to abundant punctate foci in the differentiating Type A spermatogonia, localizing to heterochromatin-rich regions (Payne and Braun, 2006). While these patterns have not been extensively evaluated in human seminiferous tubules, it is tempting to speculate that the transformation from normal primordial germ cells/gonocytes to CIS, and then subsequently to seminomas, involves the progressive upregulation of histone methyltransferase activity that results in more abundant H3K9me2 and H3K9me3 marks.

2.2 H3K27 methylation

Trimethylation of histone H3 lysine 27 (H3K27me3) is associated with transcriptional repression; this mark is established by the histone methyltransferase EZH2, a member of the Polycomb group protein family (Cao and Zhang, 2004). Similar to H3K9 methyl marks, H3K27me3 distribution is weak in CIS and abundant in seminomas (Almstrup et al., 2010). Surprisingly, EZH2 is strongly detected in the cytoplasm of CIS. Given that this enzyme normally functions in the nucleus to methylate histones, its cytoplasmic accumulation likely reflects misregulation in CIS. EZH2 is absent from embryonal carcinomas, as is H3K27me3 (Almstrup et al., 2010).

2.3 H3K4 methylation

Methylation of histone H3 lysine 4 (H3K4me1, H3K4me2, H3K4me3) is associated with transcriptional activation; H3K4me3 is established by the histone methyltransferase

Meisetz/PRDM9 (Hayashi et al., 2005). In contrast to the H3K9 and H3K27 methyl marks, H3K4me1 and H3K4me2/3 are abundant in CIS (Almstrup et al., 2010). Interestingly, the marks show opposing patterns in seminomas and non-seminomas (embryonal carcinomas), with H3K4me1 abundant in the former and weakly distributed in the latter, and H3K4me2/3 exhibiting the reverse. The significance of this observation is not clear. H3K4me2/3 appears more broadly distributed than H3K4me1 in normal human adult spermatogenic cells (Almstrup et al., 2010). As with H3K9 methyl marks, Godmann and colleagues observe H3K4me3 in both non-seminomas and seminomas (Godmann et al., 2009).

2.4 H4/H2AR3 methylation

Symmetrical dimethylation of histones H4 and H2A at arginine 3 (H4R3me2 and H2AR3me2) is associated with transcriptional repression, and is established by the complex of BLIMP1 and PRMT5 (Ancelin et al., 2006). BLIMP1 is a transcriptional repressor with an N-terminal PR-SET domain, a C-terminal acidic domain, and five zinc-finger domains; PRMT5 is a member of the protein arginine methyltransferase family. In normal fetal male germ cells of both mice and humans, H4R3me2 and H2AR3me2 marks are abundant in migratory primordial germ cells and gradually lost upon the transition to post-migratory gonocytes (Ancelin et al., 2006; Eckert, et al., 2008). In normal human adult testis, both marks are present in Type A spermatogonia, as well as round spermatids (Eckert et al., 2008). In CIS and seminomas, H4R3me2 and H2AR3me2 marks are abundant, with stronger signals detected in the seminomas. Heterogeneous, weak distribution of both marks is observed in some nonseminomatous TGCTs (embryonal carcinomas and teratomas). Dimethylation of H4R3 and H2AR3 is absent from choriocarcinomas.

2.5 EZH2

Enhancer of Zeste homolog 2 (EZH2) is a member of the Polycomb group protein family, functioning as a histone methyltransferase and adding methyl groups to H3K27 to generate H3K27me3. It is also considered to be an oncogene, shown to play a critical role in the development of breast cancer, prostate cancer, and malignant melanomas (Varambally et al., 2002; Bachmann et al., 2006). When examined in four cases of CIS, 64 seminomas, and 36 non-seminomas (9 embryonal carcinomas, 3 teratocarcinomas, and 24 mixed/combined TGCTs), *EZH2* expression showed significant downregulation when compared to normal testicular tissue (~80 vs. ~18 in CIS/TGCTs, relative normalized units), as measured by quantitative real-time RT-PCR (Hinz et al., 2009). Surprisingly, this assessment of *EZH2* mRNA conflicts with several observations of Almstrup and colleagues, who found a strong cytoplasmic distribution of EZH2 protein in CIS and abundant H3K27me3 marks in seminomas (Almstrup et al., 2010). These discrepancies could be due to the different methodologies used by the two groups (RT-PCR with oligo primers vs. immunohistochemistry with antibodies), including the processing of the specimens. As EZH2 has previously been shown to be frequently expressed in TGCTs (Bracken et al., 2003), additional studies combining both quantitative RNA and protein analysis are warranted to clarify the role of EZH2 in CIS and seminomatous/nonseminomatous TGCTs.

2.6 PRMT5

Protein arginine methyltransferase 5 forms a complex with the BLIMP1 transcriptional repressor to symmetrically dimethylate H4R3 and H2AR3. As with the histone methyl marks it generates, PRMT5 is abundant in migratory primordial germ cells and is downregulated after the cells transition to post-migratory gonocytes (Ancelin et al., 2006; Eckert, et al., 2008). In normal human adult testis, PRMT5 is present in pachytene spermatocytes and round spermatids (Eckert et al., 2008). In CIS and seminomas, PRMT5 is strongly detected in the cytoplasm and nucleus, respectively. This enzyme is also observed in the cytoplasm of embryonal carcinomas and teratomas, but is absent from choriocarcinomas. The cytoplasmic localization of PRMT5 in many of the CIS and TGCT samples, compared to the nuclear distribution seen in normal fetal germ cells, might indicate misregulation occurring as a result of the oncogenic transformation events.

2.7 JMJD3 and UTX

Jumonji domain containing 3 (JMJD3; KDM6B) and ubiquitously transcribed tetratricopeptide repeat, X chromosome (UTX; KDM6A) are histone demethylase enzymes that remove methyl groups from H3K27me2 and H3K27me3. These proteins therefore functionally oppose EZH2. In normal human adult testis, JMJD3 is weakly detected in spermatogonia and round spermatids, with stronger distribution observed in spermatocytes (Almstrup et al., 2010). UTX exhibits a similar overall pattern, with less intensity seen at each germ cell stage. In CIS, neither JMJD3 nor UTX are observed, which is concordant with high levels of EZH2 detected in these samples (Almstrup et al., 2010). In seminomatous and nonseminomatous TGCTs, JMJD3 and UTX both exhibit weak distribution at levels similar to EZH2.

2.8 HDAC1

Histone deacetylase 1 removes acetyl groups from lysine residues that are localized at the N-terminal end of histones. HDAC1, as with other members of the HDAC family, induces transcriptional repression (De Ruijter et al., 2003). In normal human adult testis, HDAC1 protein is observed in the nuclei of spermatogonia and Sertoli cells (Omisanjo et al., 2007). In both seminomatous and nonseminomatous TGCTs (embryonal carcinomas and teratomas), HDAC1 is consistently detected.

2.9 Histone modifications in Sertoli cells

HDAC1 and H3K9me3, as well as other histone modifying enzymes and modified tail residues, are present in normal human and mouse Sertoli cells (Omisanjo et al., 2007; Payne and Braun, 2006). Because Sertoli cells must maintain constant physical contact with germ cells at all stages inside each seminiferous tubule, the influence they have upon spermatogenesis is profound. Two essential growth factors that ensure the survival and maintenance of spermatogenic cells, and which are expressed by Sertoli cells, are Steel (KITL) and glial cell line-derived neurotrophic factor (GDNF). Steel activates the kit receptor (KIT) on differentiating spermatogonia in the postnatal testis, while GDNF activates associated receptors in undifferentiated spermatogonia: GDNF family receptor alpha 1 (GFRA1) and ret tyrosine kinase (RET; Sette et al., 2000; Jing et al., 1996; Viglietto et al.,

2000). Loss-of-function mutations of *Steel* and *Gdnf* in Sertoli cells deleteriously affect germ cell fate (Tajima et al., 1994; Meng et al., 2000). The loss of spermatogenic cells due to infertility or TGCTs also alters the epigenetic state of Sertoli cells, resulting in an increase in global histone H4 acetylation within the Sertoli cell nuclei of these human testes (Faure et al., 2003). In patients with seminomas and Sertoli cell-only syndrome, hyperacetylated histone H4 is observed in 70% of Sertoli cells. When Sertoli cell-specific gene targeting in mice inactivates *Sin3a*, which normally encodes an HDAC1-interacting protein, mutant testes exhibit the following: a significant reduction in spermatogonial stem cells, a progressive loss of differentiating spermatogonia, and a block in spermatid elongation, followed by extensive germ cell degeneration (Payne et al., 2010). Additionally, fewer teratomas are formed in a mouse tumor induction assay when donor germ cells from fetal *Sin3a*-mutant testes are transplanted into recipient adult testes (Payne et al, 2010). These results suggest that the epigenome in normal Sertoli cells supports a niche for spermatogonial stem cell activity, and provides a permissive microenvironment for the formation of adult TGCTs from fetal CIS. Further investigation on how Sertoli cells contribute to the development of TGCTs should increase our understanding of extrinsic factors that influence tumorigenesis.

3. Genes exhibiting promoter DNA hypermethylation

Numerous studies have shown that repetitive DNA within the human genome, consisting of Small Interspersed Nuclear Elements (SINEs), Long Interspersed Nuclear Elements (LINEs), and Long Terminal Repeats (LTRs), is globally hypomethylated in tumors (Ehrlich and Wang, 1981; Gama-Sosa et al., 1983; Dunn, 2003; Rodriguez et al., 2006). These repetitive elements are enriched in m^5C relative to the whole genome within non-tumorigenic cells, but exhibit reduced methylation relative to the genome in many cancers, including those of the breast and ovary (Narayan et al., 1998; Qu et al., 1999). One interpretation of these findings is that the loss of methylation in repetitive DNA promotes genomic instability, resulting in deletions, translocations, and chromosomal rearrangements (Eden et al., 2003; Esteller, 2008). Hypomethylated centromeric regions, for example, can contribute to aneuploidy, and the reduced methylation of satellite sequences can lead to inappropriate recombination (Hatziapostolou and Iliopoulos, 2011). Active LINEs and microsatellite DNA instability have both been discovered in TGCTs (Bratthauer and Fanning, 1992; Huddart et al., 1995). Interestingly, a recent study found that while seminomatous tumors contain both LINE1 and Alu repeats (SINE family members) in a hypomethylated state, nonseminomatous tumors exhibit hypomethylated LINE1, but methylated Alu repeats (Ushida et al., 2011).

In contrast, single-copy DNA regulatory elements of specific categories of genes undergo hypermethylation in many tumors (Estécio and Issa, 2011). CpG islands within promoter regions are usually unmethylated in non-tumorigenic cells, permitting gene transcription under the appropriate conditions (Suzuki and Bird, 2008). *De novo* methylation of CpG islands induces transcriptional silencing, often repressing tumor suppressor gene activity that creates optimal conditions for the onset and progression of most cancers. One of the first genes discovered to exhibit promoter DNA hypermethylation in tumor cells was *RB*, retinoblastoma (Sakai et al., 1991). To date, many genes identified as being susceptible to hypermethylation are known to suppress epithelial cancers, including those of the testis, prostate, lung, and colon, as well as leukemias and lymphomas (Lind et al., 2007; Wali, 2010). It is important to note that in the majority of TGCTs examined for hypermethylated gene promoters, CpG islands of most selected genes are methylated in non-seminomas, but are not appreciably methylated in seminomatous tumors (Koul et al., 2002; Honorio et al., 2003, Lind et al., 2006). In support of this finding, global detection of m^5C in CpG islands using a monoclonal antibody and immunohistochemistry revealed that the more differentiated TGCT histologies of non-seminomas (yolk sac tumors, teratomas, choriocarcinomas) exhibit hypermethylation, while the undifferentiated histology of seminomas do not show methylation (Wermann et al., 2010). Thus, it appears that in seminomas, both the repetitive DNA elements and the single-copy regulatory elements of genes are in an unmethylated state, highlighting a unique characteristic of these specific tumors. While many of the genes silenced by methylation are involved in DNA repair and the cell cycle checkpoint, others encode transcription factors, proteolytic enzymes, cell adhesion molecules, and proteins involved in various processes. Key genes that fall into each of these categories, identified to exhibit promoter DNA hypermethylation in TGCTs, will now be discussed in detail.

3.1 DNA repair/cell cycle checkpoint genes

RASSF1A

This gene encodes the Ras association domain family 1 isoform A (RASSF1A). It is one of the most prevalent hypermethylated genes across all human cancers studied (Gordon and Baksh, 2011). In addition to TGCTs, *RASSF1A* is hypermethylated in the cancers of the breast, cervix, esophagus, brain, kidney, bladder, ovary, lung and skin (Pfeifer et al., 2002; Lusher et al., 2002; Koul et al., 2002; Honorio et al., 2003; Kuroki et al., 2003; Spugnardi et al., 2003; Lind et al., 2006). RASSF1A tumor suppressor activity is important for DNA damage repair of double strand breaks and for pro-apoptotic mechanisms (Hamilton et al., 2009; Avruch et al., 2009). Four major studies detecting hypermethylated *RASSF1A* in untreated TGCTs have been published to date, with conflicting results for seminomas. Koul and colleagues reported that of the seminomatous and nonseminomatous TGCTs they examined, nearly all of the hypermethylated CpG islands were observed in non-seminomas (frequencies of ~100% in yolk sac tumors, ~45% in embryonal carcinomas, ~22% in teratomas, and ~9% in mixed/combined tumors); only 1 of 29 seminomas exhibited hypermethylated *RASSF1A* (Koul et al., 2002). In their examination of TGCTs, Honorio et al. found hypermethylated CpG islands in 15 of 18 (83%) non-seminomas, with frequencies of 80% (4/5) in yolk sac tumors, 60% (3/5) in embryonal carcinomas, 100% (5/5) in teratomas, and 100% in two choriocarcinomas and one mixed tumor; 4 of 10 (40%) seminomas exhibited *RASSF1A* hypermethylation, distinguishing these results from the previous study (Honorio et al., 2003). Lind and colleagues, meanwhile, observed elevated methylation in 10 of 35 (28.6%) nonseminomatous TGCTs and in 0 of 19 seminomas (Lind et al., 2006). The frequencies in the non-seminomas were: 50% (3/6) in yolk sac tumors, 37.5% (6/16) in embryonal carcinomas, 77.8% (7/9) in teratomas, and 100% in one choriocarcinoma. In contrast, Tian et al. recently reported that both seminomatous and nonseminomatous tumors contained equivalent frequencies of hypermethylated *RASSF1A* CpG islands (~78.6%), with an average of 13/16 CpG sites in a methylated state as measured by sodium bisulfite sequencing (Tian et al., 2011). In an earlier study, Kawakami and colleagues did not detect the hypermethylation of *RASSF1A*, or any other gene they examined, in any of the TGCTs under investigation (Kawakami et al., 2003). Thus, from all of these studies it appears that *RASSF1A* is hypermethylated at a frequency of up to 100% in yolk sac tumors, teratomas, choriocarcinomas, and up to 60% in embryonal carcinomas, but exhibits divergent methylation patterns in seminomas. Further characterization of *RASSF1A* in seminomas is needed to address these discrepancies. Interestingly, when Koul and colleagues examined 39 cisplatin-resistant and 31 cisplatin-sensitive non-seminomas, *RASSF1A* exhibited a much higher frequency of methylation in the cisplatin-resistant group (52%) than in the cisplatin-sensitive group (28%), though the sample size was too small for statistical significance (Koul et al., 2004). The methylation status of the *RASSF1A* promoter might therefore be a useful prognostic indicator of nonseminomatous tumor sensitivity to cisplatin, and could allow for the adjustment of chemotherapy treatment strategy accordingly. Finally, it has been shown that hypermethylated *RASSF1A* CpG islands are detected in the cell-free circulating serum DNA of TGCT patients at a frequency of ~47% (Ellinger et al., 2009). This method of detection could provide an additional benefit to existing parameters in the clinic.

MGMT

This gene encodes O-6-methylguanine-DNA methyltransferase (MGMT), which provides defense against the mutagenic effects of O-6-methylguanine (alkylation adduct) in DNA and potential G-to-A transition mutations. MGMT repairs the O-6 position of guanine in DNA by transferring the alkyl group from this position to a cysteine residue within the structure of the protein (Mitra, 2007). The *MGMT* promoter is hypermethylated in glioblastomas, hepatocellular carcinomas, colorectal, esophageal, and lung cancers, as well as in TGCTs (Cao et al., 2009; Zhang et al., 2003; Ahlquist et al., 2008; Baumann et al., 2006; Wolf et al., 2001; Smith-Sørensen et al., 2002; Koul et al., 2002; Honorio et al., 2003; Koul et al., 2004). Smith-Sørensen and colleagues identified hypermethylated CpG islands in both seminomatous tumors (24%, 8/33) and nonseminomatous tumors (69%, 24/35), while the groups of Koul and Honorio found *MGMT* hypermethylation only in non-seminomas (frequencies of ~25% in yolk sac tumors, ~45% in embryonal carcinomas, ~30% in teratomas, and ~9% in mixed/combined tumors for Koul et al.); 44% of non-seminomas exhibited hypermethylated *MGMT* for Honorio and colleagues (Smith-Sørensen et al., 2002; Koul et al., 2002; Honorio et al., 2003). In contrast to *RASSF1A*, Koul et al. found that *MGMT* was hypermethylated more often in cisplatin-sensitive non-seminomas (31%) than in cisplatin-resistant tumors (13%), though the P-value was not significant (Koul et al., 2004). Compared to the hypermethylation of *RASSF1A* and all other genes examined in TGCTs, *MGMT* exhibited the highest frequency of hypermethylation in seminomas (11%, 8 of 72 combined from all three studies). Given the overall small sample sizes and discrepancies reported among the groups, it would be worth conducting a larger study examining *RASSF1A* and *MGMT* hypermethylation in seminomas to more accurately conclude whether the CpG islands of these genes might be the exception to the overall trend of unmethylated cytosine in seminoma DNA.

BRCA1

Breast cancer 1 encodes a multi-faceted protein involved in numerous cellular functions: DNA damage repair, cell cycle checkpoint, centrosome duplication, transcriptional regulation, and many others (Deng and Brodie, 2000). Hypermethylated *BRCA1* is observed in a variety of cancers, including breast, ovary, bladder, lung, and testis (Rice et al., 2000; Bianco et al., 2000; Cabello et al., 2011; Wang et al., 2008; Koul et al., 2002). Koul and colleagues reported that of the seminomatous and nonseminomatous TGCTs they examined, nearly all of the hypermethylated CpG islands were observed in non-seminomas (frequencies of ~49% in yolk sac tumors, and equivalent percentages in embryonal carcinomas, teratomas, and mixed/combined tumors, 20-24%); only 1 of 29 seminomas exhibited hypermethylated *BRCA1* (Koul et al., 2002). No differences were observed between cisplatin-sensitive (31%) and –resistant (30%) non-seminomas with respect to CpG island methylation (Koul et al., 2004).

FANCF

Fanconi anemia, complementation group F encodes a DNA repair protein that supports post-replication repair, cell cycle checkpoint function, and maintenance of normal chromosome stability (Léveillé et al., 2004). *FANCF* is hypermethylated in cervical and ovarian cancers, as well as TGCTs (Narayan et al., 2004; Taniguchi et al., 2003; Koul et al., 2004). Koul and colleagues examined CpG island methylation only in nonseminomatous tumors, and found the overall frequency to be 5.7%. No differences were observed between cisplatin-sensitive (7%) and –resistant (6%) non-seminomas with respect to hypermethylated *FANCF* (Koul et al., 2004).

XPA

Xeroderma pigmentosum, complementation group A encodes a zinc finger protein that participates in the initial step of DNA excision repair (de Vries and van Steeg, 1996). XPA guards against the harmful effects of UV-B radiation and chemical compounds that would otherwise impair DNA replication and RNA transcription. While *XPA* expression is diminished in some colorectal cancers, CpG methylation has only been observed in one nonseminomatous TGCT (Yu et al., 2006; Lind et al., 2006). Lind and colleagues found that one of 6 yolk sac tumors exhibited hypermethylated *XPA*; no methylation was detected in any of 16 embryonal carcinomas, 9 teratomas, 1 choriocarcinoma, 3 mixed/combined tumors, and 20 seminomas (Lind et al., 2006). Thus, it appears that *XPA* is not appreciably methylated in either seminomas or non-seminomas.

MLH1

mutL homolog 1 (a homolog of the *E. coli* DNA mismatch repair gene *mutL*) encodes a protein that forms a component of the post-replicative DNA mismatch repair system. MLH1 is involved in DNA damage signaling, inducing cell cycle arrest and apoptosis under certain conditions (Buermeyer et al., 1999). The *MLH1* promoter is hypermethylated in numerous cancers, including colorectal, gastric, and endometrial carcinomas, and tumors of the breast, ovary, and testis (Herman et al., 1998; Leung et al., 1999; Esteller et al., 1998; Murata et al., 2002; Strathdee et al., 1999; Koul et al., 2002; Olasz et al., 2005). Koul and colleagues reported that of the seminomatous and nonseminomatous TGCTs they examined, nearly all of the hypermethylated CpG islands were observed in non-seminomas (no methylation detected in yolk sac tumors or teratomas, and frequencies of <10% in embryonal carcinomas and mixed/combined tumors); only 1 of 29 seminomas exhibited hypermethylated *MLH1* (Koul et al., 2002). Olasz et al. found an overall methylation frequency of 21.6% in the TGCTs they examined, yet only 1 in 15 samples from refractory tumors showed CpG hypermethylation (Olasz et al., 2005). Unlike what has been observed in familiar colorectal cancer, no correlation exists between *MLH1* methylation status and microsatellite instability in TGCTs (Herman et al., 1998; Olasz et al., 2005). No relationship is seen between the clinical outcome of TGCTs and *MLH1* hypermethylation, dampening its prospect as a potential biomarker.

APC

adenomatous polyposis coli encodes a tumor suppressor protein that antagonizes Wnt signaling. APC is also critical for cell migration and adhesion, transcriptional activation, DNA repair, and apoptosis (Senda et al., 2007). Hypermethylated *APC* is observed in many cancers, including colorectal, esophageal, breast, lung, prostate, and testis (Hiltunen et al., 1997; Kawakami et al., 2000; Virmani et al., 2001; Yegnasubramanian et al., 2004; Koul et al., 2002; Honorio et al., 2003). Koul and colleagues found an overall CpG methylation frequency of 9.8% in the nonseminomatous TGCTs they examined (~100% in yolk sac tumors, ~12% in teratomas, and ~3% in mixed/combined tumors; no methylation seen in embryonal carcinomas or seminomas), while Honorio et al. detected *APC* hypermethylation in 29% of non-seminomas (Koul et al., 2002; Honorio et al., 2003). No differences were observed between cisplatin-sensitive (24%) and -resistant (29%) non-seminomas with respect to hypermethylated *APC* (Koul et al., 2004). It was also recently shown that hypermethylated CpG islands of *APC* are detected in the cell-free circulating serum DNA of TGCT patients at a frequency of ~58% (Ellinger et al., 2009).

FHIT

fragile histidine triad gene encodes an enzyme, diadenosine 5',5'''-P1,P3-triphosphate hydrolase, that is involved in purine metabolism. It also promotes genomic integrity through DNA damage response and DNA repair mechanisms (Saldivar et al., 2010). *FHIT* is one of the most frequent targets of allele deletion in tumors, and is hypermethylated in cancers of the lung, cervix, liver, and testis (Hsu et al., 2007; Ki et al., 2008; Iyer et al., 2010; Koul et al., 2002; Honorio et al., 2003). Koul and colleagues observed *FHIT* hypermethylation at an overall frequency of 6.5% in non-seminomas (~49% in yolk sac tumors, ~8% in embryonal carcinomas, ~2% in teratomas, and ~3% in mixed/combined tumors), while Honorio et al. detected CpG methylation in 29% of nonseminomatous tumors (Koul et al., 2002; Honorio et al., 2003). No differences were observed between cisplatin-sensitive (7%) and -resistant (6%) non-seminomas with respect to hypermethylated *FHIT* (Koul et al., 2004).

CDKN2A

cyclin-dependent kinase inhibitor 2A generates multiple transcript variants that differ in their first exons. One of the transcripts contains an alternate open reading frame (ARF), yielding a protein that stabilizes tumor suppressor p53 through the sequestration of MDM2 (Gjerset, 2006). CDKN2A can also induce cell cycle arrest in G1 and G2, and promote apoptosis. *CDKN2A* hypermethylation in the forms of *p14(ARF)* and *p16(INK)* has been detected in numerous cancers, including those of the colon, stomach, kidney, uterus, ovary, and testis (Esteller et al., 2001; Chaubert et al., 1997). Variable results have been shown for TGCTs. Chaubert and colleagues reported the presence of hypermethylated *CDKN2A* in 13 of 26 (50%) TGCTs using the method of PCR amplification after *HpaII* enzyme digestion

(Chaubert et al., 1997). The groups of Smith-Sørensen, Honorio, and Kawakami, in contrast, were not able to detect methylated CpG islands of *CDKN2A* when examined by methylation-specific PCR (Smith-Sørensen et al., 2002; Honorio et al., 2003; Kawakami et al., 2003). Differing experimental strategies might explain this discrepancy. Hypermethylation of *p14(ARF)* and *p16(INK)* was recently observed in the cell-free circulating serum DNA of TGCT patients at a frequency of ~53% (Ellinger et al., 2009).

3.2 Transcription factor genes

NANOG

This gene encodes an important regulator of pluripotency maintenance in the inner cell mass of blastocyst-stage embryos and in undifferentiated embryonic stem cells. NANOG prevents differentiation into mesoderm by interacting with SMAD1 and blocking the recruitment of co-activators in that signaling pathway (Suzuki et al., 2006). Migratory primordial germ cells express *NANOG*, but upon the differentiation of male germ cells into fetal gonocytes and neonatal spermatogonia, *NANOG* is downregulated (Gaskell et al., 2004). Thus, normal juvenile and adult male germ cells do not express *NANOG*. Interestingly, Nettersheim et al. detected hypomethylated *NANOG*, and corresponding protein, in all seminomas and embryonal carcinomas (undifferentiated non-seminomas) they obtained from TGCT patients (Nettersheim et al., 2011). In contrast, all differentiated non-seminomas (yolk sac tumors, teratomas, and choriocarcinomas) exhibited CpG hypermethylation and an absence of NANOG protein. Similarly, normal adult spermatogonia contain hypermethylated *NANOG*, supporting the prevailing hypothesis that seminomas are derived from gonocyte precursors in the fetal gonad (Nettersheim et al., 2011). Thus, differences within the state of TGCT differentiation correlate with the extent of *NANOG* hypermethylation.

HIC1

hypermethylated in cancer 1 encodes a transcriptional repressor protein that functionally interacts with p53 to suppress the development of cancer throughout aging (Chen et al., 2005). The *HIC1* promoter is hypermethylated in many cancers, including those of the breast, cervix, and testis (Fujii et al., 1998; Dong et al., 2001; Koul et al., 2002). Koul and colleagues observed *HIC1* hypermethylation only in non-seminomas (frequencies of ~100% in yolk sac tumors, ~35% in embryonal carcinomas, ~21% in teratomas, and ~9% in mixed/combined tumors). None of 29 seminomas exhibited hypermethylated *HIC1* (Koul et al., 2002). *HIC1* also exhibited a much higher frequency of methylation in the cisplatin-resistant group (47%) than in the cisplatin-sensitive group (24%), though the sample size was too small for statistical significance (Koul et al., 2004). Like *RASSF1A*, the methylation status of the *HIC1* promoter could be a useful prognostic indicator of nonseminomatous tumor sensitivity to cisplatin.

HOXA9

homeobox A9 encodes a transcription factor that regulates differentiation and morphogenesis, and is important for hematopoiesis (Lawrence et al., 1997). Hypermethylated *HOXA9* has been reported for ovarian carcinomas, oral squamous cell carcinomas, lung cancer, liver cancer, and TGCTs (Wu et al., 2007; Guerrero-Preston et al., 2011; Hwang et al., 2011; Feng et al., 2010; Lind et al., 2006). Lind and colleagues observed *HOXA9* hypermethylation only in nonseminomatous tumors, in 9 of 35 samples (detected in yolk sac tumors, teratomas, and one choriocarcinoma; Lind et al., 2006).

HOXB5

homeobox B5 encodes a transcription factor involved in lung and gut development, regulating differentiation and morphogenesis, and providing specific positional identities on the anterior-posterior axis (Volpe et al., 1997; Fu et al., 2003). Hypermethylated *HOXB5* has been reported for ovarian carcinomas and TGCTs (Wu et al., 2007; Lind et al., 2006). Lind and colleagues observed *HOXB5* hypermethylation only in nonseminomatous tumors, in 5 of 35 samples (detected exclusively in teratomas; Lind et al., 2006).

RARB

retinoic acid receptor, beta encodes a nuclear receptor that binds to retinoic acid, heterodimerizing with the retinoid x receptor and regulating transcriptional activity though retinoic acid response elements located in target genes (Dollé, 2009). *RARB* hypermethylation has been detected in numerous cancers, including those of the cervix, prostate, lung, bladder, and testis (Narayan et al., 2003; Singal et al., 2004; Feng et al., 2008; Cabello et al., 2011; Koul et al., 2002; Honorio et al., 2003). The groups of Koul and Honorio found *RARB* hypermethylation only in non-seminomas (frequencies of ~49% in yolk sac tumors, ~15% in embryonal carcinomas, and ~5% in teratomas for Koul et al.); only 5% of non-seminomas exhibited hypermethylated *RARB* for Honorio and colleagues (Koul et al., 2002; Honorio et al., 2003). Koul et al. also found that *RARB* was hypermethylated more often in cisplatin-sensitive non-seminomas (14%) than in cisplatin-resistant tumors (0%), with a P-value of 0.05 (Koul et al., 2004).

EMX2

empty spiracles homeobox 2 encodes a transcription factor that regulates neuroblast proliferation, migration and differentiation, patterns the forebrain, and defines cortical territories (Cecchi, 2002). In the urogenital system, *EMX2* is expressed in epithelial cells and is negatively regulated by HOXA10 (Troy et al., 2003). Hypermethylated *EMX2* has been reported for lung cancer and TGCTs (Okamoto et al., 2010; Lind et al., 2006). Lind and colleagues found that one of 6 yolk sac tumors exhibited hypermethylated *EMX2;* no methylation was detected in any of 16 embryonal carcinomas, 9 teratomas, 1 choriocarcinoma, 3 mixed/combined tumors, and 20 seminomas (Lind et al., 2006). Thus, it appears that *EMX2* is not appreciably methylated in either seminomas or non-seminomas.

MSX1

msh homeobox 1 encodes a member of the muscle segment homeobox gene family. Functioning as a transcriptional repressor, MSX1 influences limb pattern formation and craniofacial development (Alappat et al., 2003). Hypermethylated *MSX1* has been reported for acute lymphoblastic leukemia, and cancers of the breast, lung, colon, prostate, and testis (Dunwell et al., 2009; Shames et al., 2006; Lind et al., 2006). Lind and colleagues found that one of 6 yolk sac tumors exhibited hypermethylated *MSX1;* no methylation was detected in any of 16 embryonal carcinomas, 9 teratomas, 1 choriocarcinoma, 3 mixed/combined tumors, and 20 seminomas (Lind et al., 2006). Thus, it appears that *MSX1* is not appreciably methylated in either seminomas or non-seminomas.

RUNX3

runt-related transcription factor 3 encodes a member of the runt domain-containing family of transcription factors that binds to core sequences found in a number of enhancers and promoters (Otto et al., 2003). The *RUNX3* promoter is hypermethylated in many cancers, including those of the lung, liver, colon, bladder, breast, and testis (Li et al., 2004; Xiao and Liu, 2004; Goel et al., 2004; Kim et al., 2005; Hwang et al., 2007; Kato et al., 2003; Lind et al., 2006). Interestingly, Kato and colleagues reported that while 8 of 10 infantile yolk sac tumors exhibited *RUNX3* hypermethylation (specimens obtained from pediatric patients), 0 of 12 adult nonseminomatous TGCTs contained methylated *RUNX3*, despite 7 of the 11 mixed/combined TGCTs containing yolk sac tumors (Kato et al., 2003). Similarly, Lind et al. found that only one of 6 adult yolk sac tumors exhibited hypermethylated *RUNX3*, and no methylation was detected in any of 49 other adult non-seminomas (16 embryonal carcinomas, 9 teratomas, 1 choriocarcinoma, 3 mixed/combined tumors, and 20 seminomas; Lind et al., 2006). These observations strongly suggest that distinct epigenetic dysregulatory mechanisms occur in pediatric, but not adult yolk sac tumors, and that *RUNX3* is not appreciably methylated in either seminomatous or nonseminomatous adult TGCTs.

3.3 Proteolysis genes

PRSS21

protease, serine, 21 encodes a member of the trypsin family of serine proteases that uses the hydroxyl group of serine to cleave target peptide bonds involving the carboxyl group of lysine or arginine (Rawlings and Barrett, 1994). *PRSS21* is thought to regulate proteolytic events associated with male germ cell maturation, as it is expressed highly only in normal testis, and its hypermethylation and transcriptional repression have been observed in TGCTs (Manton et al., 2005; Kempkensteffen et al., 2006). Manton and colleagues reported that the majority of CpG islands were methylated in both seminomatous (86%, 3 samples) and nonseminomatous (87%, 5 samples) tumors (Manton et al., 2005). While Kempkensteffen et al. found the overall level of hypermethylation lower in seminomas than in non-seminomas, the levels were still significantly higher when compared to normal testicular tissue (Kempkensteffen et al., 2006). Thus, *PRSS21* appears to show the most extensive hypermethylation of any gene examined to date in seminomas, and might therefore be a useful biomarker for early detection of these tumors in the clinic, especially if detected in the cell-free circulating serum DNA.

TIMP3

tissue inhibitor of metalloproteinase 3 encodes a protein that inhibits matrix metalloproteinases, enzymes that degrade components of the extracellular matrix (Apte et al., 1995). *TIMP3* hypermethylation has been detected in numerous cancers, including those of the kidney, colon, breast, brain, lung, and testis (Esteller et al., 2001; Koul et al., 2002). Koul and colleagues, however, observed an overall frequency of hypermethylation of just 3.3% in non-seminomas, with detection of methylated CpG islands limited to embryonal carcinomas and mixed/combined tumors (Koul et al., 2002). No hypermethylation was seen in seminomas. Therefore, compared to other genes, *TIMP3* does not appear to be as extensively hypermethylated in non-seminomas.

3.4 Cell adhesion genes

CDH1

cadherin 1 encodes a calcium dependent cell-cell adhesion glycoprotein highly expressed in epithelial tissues, E-cadherin, that is comprised of five extracellular cadherin repeats, a transmembrane region, and a highly conserved cytoplasmic tail. Mutations in *CDH1* that disrupt the adhesive properties of E-cadherin occur in some breast and gastric carcinomas (Hirohashi, 1998). *CDH1* hypermethylation is also detected in many cancers, including leukemia and those of the esophagus, breast, prostate, and testis (Esteller et al., 2001; Koul et al., 2002; Honorio et al., 2003). Koul and colleagues reported that of the seminomatous and nonseminomatous TGCTs they examined, the majority of hypermethylated CpG islands were observed in non-seminomas (frequencies of <10% in embryonal carcinomas, teratomas, and mixed/combined tumors); only 1 of 29 seminomas exhibited hypermethylated *CDH1* (Koul et al., 2002). Honorio et al. detected an overall methylation frequency of 11% in non-seminomas (Honorio et al., 2003). No differences were observed between cisplatin-sensitive (3%) and -resistant (6%) non-seminomas with respect to hypermethylated *CDH1* (Koul et al., 2004).

CDH13

cadherin 13 encodes a calcium dependent cell-cell adhesion glycoprotein highly expressed in heart tissues, H-cadherin, that is comprised of five extracellular cadherin repeats, a transmembrane region, but unlike other cadherins, lacks the highly conserved cytoplasmic tail. The *CDH13* promoter is hypermethylated in numerous cancers, including chronic myeloid leukemia and those of the breast, lung, bladder, and testis (Roman-Gomez et al., 2003; Toyooka et al., 2001; Maruyama et al., 2001; Honorio et al., 2003; Lind et al., 2006). Honorio and colleagues reported an overall frequency of hypermethylated *CDH13* in 12% of non-seminomas, while Lind et al. detected hypermethylation in 9% of nonseminomatous (2 of 16 embryonal carcinomas; 0 of 9 teratomas) and 6% (1/17) of seminomatous TGCTs (Honorio et al., 2003; Lind et al., 2006). Despite the small sample size, *CDH13* hypermethylation was observed in the more undifferentiated TGCTs and not in the more highly differentiated non-seminomas, distinguishing this gene from most others that have been described here.

3.5 Genes involved in other processes

SCGB3A1 (extracellular/cytokine)

secretoglobin, family 3A, member 1 encodes a secreted protein, formerly called *high in normal 1* (*HIN1*), which has tumor suppressor activity, although the exact function of the protein is unknown. *SCGB3A1* is highly expressed in the lung and trachea of humans and mice, with additional expression in a species-dependent manner (Tomita and Kimura, 2008). Hypermethylated *SCGB3A1* has been reported for cancers of the nasopharynx, breast, lung, prostate, pancreas, stomach, and testis, among others (Wong et al., 2003; Fackler et al., 2003; Krop et al., 2004; Gong et al., 2011; Lind et al., 2006). Lind and colleagues observed *SCGB3A1* hypermethylation in 19 of 35 non-seminomas (frequencies of ~100% in choriocarcinomas, ~75% in teratomas, ~47% in yolk sac tumors, and ~35% in embryonal carcinomas); no methylation was detected in seminomas (Lind et al., 2006).

SORBS1 (glucose transport)

sorbin and SH3 domain containing 1 encodes a protein involved in tyrosine phosphorylation of c-Abl, via an interaction with the insulin receptor, and is required for insulin-stimulated glucose transport (Lin et al., 2001). Lind and colleagues reported *SORBS1* hypermethylation in 1 of 20 seminomatous TGCTs examined, with no detection in non-seminomas (0/35; Lind et al., 2006). Given the sample size, additional studies will be necessary to conclusively determine whether this gene is a useful biomarker for TGCTs.

GSTP1 (metabolic process)

glutathione S-transferase, pi 1 encodes an enzyme important for detoxification by catalyzing the conjugation of hydrophobic and electrophilic compounds with reduced glutathione (Strange et al., 2001). The GST family is categorized into four classes: alpha, mu, pi, and theta. *GSTP1* hypermethylation is observed in many cancers, including those of the liver, kidney, breast, lung, esophagus, brain, and colon (Esteller et al., 2001). The groups of Kawakami and Honorio did not find hypermethylated *GSTP1* in any of their seminomatous or nonseminomatous TGCT samples, but Koul et al. reported *GSTP1* hypermethylation in 1 of 29 seminomas (none in non-seminomas) and Ellinger et al. detected CpG island methylation in the cell-free circulating serum DNA of TGCT patients at a frequency of ~25% (Koul et al., 2002; Kawakami et al., 2003; Honorio et al., 2003; Ellinger et al., 2009). The TGCT patients had seminomas (N=36) as well as non-seminomas (N=37), and the hypermethylation frequency observed by Ellinger and colleagues was equivalent between the two groups (Ellinger et al., 2009). Clearly, additional studies will be necessary to determine why discrepancies exist between not observing *GSTP1* hypermethylation in the majority of TGCT samples and frequently observing it in the cell-free serum DNA of TGCT patients.

PTGS2 (oxidation-reduction)

prostaglandin-endoperoxidase synthase 2 encodes a key enzyme in prostaglandin biosynthesis, also known as COX2, which acts as both a dioxygenase and a peroxidase. Two isozymes of PTGS exist, the constitutive PTGS1 and the inducible PTGS2, which differ in their regulation of expression and tissue distribution. This gene encodes the inducible isozyme, and is misregulated in many cancers (Rizzo, 2011). Hypermethylated *PTGS2* has been reported for gliomas, gastric carcinomas, prostate cancer, and breast cancer, among others (Uhlmann et al., 2003; Yu et al., 2003; Yegnasubramanian et al., 2004; Chow et al., 2005). Ellinger and colleagues detected *PTGS2* CpG island hypermethylation in the cell-free circulating serum DNA of TGCT patients at a frequency of ~45%; no differences were observed between patients with seminomas and those with non-seminomas (Ellinger et al., 2009). It remains to be seen whether a similar frequency of hypermethylation is observed directly in TGCT specimens. Currently, the cell-free serum-based detection of hypermethylated *PTGS2*, like *RASSF1A*, *APC*, *CDKN2A* and *GSTP1*, could provide additional benefits to existing parameters in the clinic.

NME2 (phosphorylation)

non-metastatic cells 2, protein (NM23B) expressed in (official gene name) encodes a protein that, together with the product of *NME1*, forms the hexamer nucleoside diphosphate kinase (Postel et al., 2002). Koul and colleagues reported *NME2* CpG hypermethylation in one embryonal carcinoma sample (Koul et al., 2002), but no other known observations in

TGCTs or other cancers have been published, raising the uncertainty over the significance of this discovery.

4. DNA methyltransferases

DNA methylation is established by the coordinated activity of enzymes known as DNA methyltransferases (DNMTs). The mammalian DNMT family consists of DNMT1, DNMT3A, DNMT3B, and DNMT3L, and is responsible for the generation, acquisition, and maintenance of methylated cytosines residing in CpG dinucleotides (Jurkowska et al., 2010). DNMT3A and DNMT3B are *de novo* methyltransferases, while DNMT1 is a maintenance methyltransferase, required to preserve the methylated status of the DNA. Levels of DNMTs are increased in numerous cancers, accounting for the hypermethylation of CpG islands observed in the promoters of many genes. Thus, DNMTs are promising targets for the design of new anti-cancer therapeutics.

4.1 DNMT1

DNA methyltransferase 1 is responsible for the maintenance of the DNA methylation status in CpG dinucleotides (Bestor et al., 1988). Hypermethylation of CpG islands in gene promoters, as Section 3 in this chapter extensively describes, is associated with the transcriptional silencing of tumor suppressors and other genes in many cancers, including TGCTs. Omisanjo and colleagues examined the expression of DNMT1 mRNA and protein in TGCTs to determine whether *DNMT1* is upregulated. In normal human adult testis, *DNMT1* mRNA is expressed in spermatogonia, pachytene spermatocytes, and round spermatids, as measured by *in situ* hybridization; the protein is nuclear in spermatogonia, cytoplasmic in round spermatids, and interestingly, is not detected in pachytene spermatocytes (Omisanjo et al., 2007). In non-seminomas (8 embryonal carcinomas and 8 teratomas), both mRNA and protein are detected, with a stronger signal observed in the embryonal carcinomas. Neither mRNA nor protein are detected in seminomas (0/16; Omisanjo et al., 2007). These differential TGCT expression patterns of *DNMT1* were also found using RNA microarray analysis and quantitative real-time RT-PCR, showing significantly upregulated transcript levels in embryonal carcinomas, but low levels in seminomas (Biermann et al., 2007). In contrast, semi-quantitative RT-PCR analysis performed by Ishii and colleagues showed no difference in *DNMT1* expression between control tissue and either seminomatous or nonseminomatous TGCTs (Ishii et al., 2007). DNA methyltransferase inhibitors, such as 5-aza-2′-deoxycytidine, have been shown to reactivate silenced tumor suppressor genes in treated cancer cells, implying that DNMTs are both necessary and sufficient to maintain hypermethylated CpG islands in many tumors.

4.2 DNMT3A

DNA methyltransferase 3A is responsible for the *de novo* transfer of methyl groups to CpG dinucleotides. DNMT3A catalyzes the transfer of a methyl group from S-adenosyl-methionine to the 5′ position of cytosine in DNA (Okano et al., 1999). Studies in mice have shown that DNMT3A is essential for imprinting, as well as for spermatogenesis (Kaneda et al., 2004). Ishii and colleagues recently examined the expression of DNMT3A mRNA and protein in TGCTs, known to exhibit hypermethylated CpG islands in numerous genes, to determine whether *DNMT3A* is upregulated. Semi-quantitative RT-PCR analysis revealed that *DNMT3A* and its isoform, *DNMT3A2*, are significantly overexpressed in seminomas as well as non-seminomas (embryonal carcinomas, teratomas, choriocarcinomas, yolk sac tumors; Ishii et al., 2007). Protein analysis by immunoblot revealed that the DNMT3A2 isoform is exhibited several times higher than control levels in both seminomatous and nonseminomatous TGCTs (Ishii et al., 2007). Thus, the upregulation of *DNMT3A2* appears to generate higher amounts of protein, and seems to be tumor cell-specific. Ishii et al. then examined the methylation levels of CpG-rich regions in the *DNMT3A* gene, and found more unmethylated *DNMT3A* CpG dinucleotides in seminomas than in adjacent non-tumor tissue (Ishii et al., 2007). Overexpression of *DNMT3A* in TGCTs therefore appears to result from the hypomethylation of CpG islands in key regulatory regions, allowing inappropriate transcription to occur.

4.3 DNMT3B

DNA methyltransferase 3B is responsible for the *de novo* transfer of methyl groups to CpG dinucleotides. DNMT3B catalyzes the transfer of a methyl group from S-adenosyl-methionine to the 5′ position of cytosine in DNA (Okano et al., 1999). Beyrouthy and colleagues recently examined the protein expression of DNMT3B in embryonal carcinoma cell lines to determine whether they exhibit higher protein levels than in normal tissues or somatic tumors. Western blot analysis revealed that DNMT3B is significantly overexpressed in embryonal carcinoma cell lines when compared to all other cell types (Beyrouthy et al., 2009). Three earlier microarray studies reported upregulated *DNMT3B* mRNA in non-seminomas (primarily embryonal carcinomas), but not in seminomas when compared to non-cancerous controls (Almstrup et al., 2005; Korkola et al., 2005; Skotheim et al., 2005). In contrast, Ishii et al. found no significant difference in *DNMT3B* expression between control tissue and either seminomatous or nonseminomatous TGCTs, which were mostly teratomas, choriocarcinomas, and yolk sac tumors (Ishii et al., 2007). This difference in TGCT sample type could explain the discrepancy in the results; clearly *DNMT3B* appears to be overexpressed in embryonal carcinomas. Furthermore, knockdown of *DNMT3B* reverses 5-aza-2′-deoxycytidine hypersensitivity in both cisplatin-sensitive and cisplatin-resistant embryonal carcinoma cells (Beyrouthy et al., 2009). While cisplatin sensitivity itself is not affected by *DNMT3B* expression, 5-aza-2′-deoxycytidine hypersensitivity in embryonal carcinoma cells appears to be dependent on *DNMT3B* expression, regardless of whether the cells are sensitive or resistant to cisplatin.

5. Clinical applications

When compared to many other cancers, a remarkable aspect in the majority of TGCTs is the high curability rate using cisplatin-based chemotherapy in combination with radiation therapy. However, up to 30% of metastatic germ cell tumors of the testis are refractory to cisplatin treatment and can lead to mortality. As discussed earlier, hypermethylation of CpG islands in the promoters of two genes, *RASSF1A* and *HIC1*, has been observed in cisplatin-resistant tumors at a frequency of approximately 50%, while promoter hypermethylation for *MGMT* and *RARB* has been detected at higher frequencies in cisplatin-sensitive vs. chemoresistant tumors (Koul *et al.*, 2004). Recent investigation into the use of DNA demethylating agent 5-azacytidine in TCam-2 cells as a method to decrease cisplatin resistance has shown promising results (Wermann *et al.*, 2010). Drugs that target DNMTs are currently in use in clinical trials, such as 5-aza-2′-deoxycytidine for treating myelodysplastic syndromes (Müller-Thomas et al., 2009), and newer drugs are under development.

6. Conclusion

A greater understanding of the role of histone modifications, histone modifying enzymes, genes exhibiting promoter DNA hypermethylation, and DNA methyltransferases in adult TGCTs should yield potentially useful biomarkers to aid in early detection, as well as new methods of treatment to overcome chemotherapy-resistant tumors. The presence of hypermethylated *RASSF1A, APC, CDKN2A, GSTP1,* and *PTGS2* in the cell-free serum DNA of TGCT patients raises the important question of how early in the tumorigenic process these markers could be detected at interpretable levels. Optimizing this strategy of identifying potential TGCTs before they develop to the extent of requiring aggressive chemotherapy and radiation treatment will be an important endeavor during the next decade. Because some metastatic TGCTs are refractory to cisplatin-based chemotherapy, searching for an alternative treatment regimen for these tumors is equally important. The potential use of 5-azacytidine, or similar DNMT inhibitors, in overcoming cisplatin resistance holds promise for such cases. Further investigation of epigenetic modifications in TGCTs at the bench and in the clinic will address these goals.

7. Acknowledgment

The author is grateful to the members of his lab, Jessica Huszar, Shannon Gallagher, and Amber Kofman, for many thoughtful discussions during the writing of this chapter. Financial support is provided by the Medical Research Institute Council of Children's Memorial Hospital.

8. References

Ahlquist, T., Lind, G. E., Costa, V. L., Meling, G. I., Vatn, M., Hoff, G. S., Rognum, T. O., Skotheim, R. I., Thiis-Evensen, E. and Lothe, R. A. (2008) 'Gene methylation profiles of normal mucosa, and benign and malignant colorectal tumors identify early onset markers', *Molecular cancer* 7: 94.

Alappat, S., Zhang, Z. Y. and Chen, Y. P. (2003) 'Msx homeobox gene family and craniofacial development', *Cell research* 13(6): 429-42.

Almstrup, K., Hoei-Hansen, C. E., Nielsen, J. E., Wirkner, U., Ansorge, W., Skakkebaek, N. E., Rajpert-De Meyts, E. and Leffers, H. (2005) 'Genome-wide gene expression profiling of testicular carcinoma in situ progression into overt tumours', *British journal of cancer* 92(10): 1934-41.

Almstrup, K., Nielsen, J. E., Mlynarska, O., Jansen, M. T., Jorgensen, A., Skakkebaek, N. E. and Rajpert-De Meyts, E. (2010) 'Carcinoma in situ testis displays permissive chromatin modifications similar to immature foetal germ cells', *British journal of cancer* 103(8): 1269-76.

Ancelin, K., Lange, U. C., Hajkova, P., Schneider, R., Bannister, A. J., Kouzarides, T. and Surani, M. A. (2006) 'Blimp1 associates with Prmt5 and directs histone arginine methylation in mouse germ cells', *Nature cell biology* 8(6): 623-30.

Apte, S. S., Olsen, B. R. and Murphy, G. (1995) 'The gene structure of tissue inhibitor of metalloproteinases (TIMP)-3 and its inhibitory activities define the distinct TIMP gene family', *The Journal of biological chemistry* 270(24): 14313-8.

Avruch, J., Xavier, R., Bardeesy, N., Zhang, X. F., Praskova, M., Zhou, D. and Xia, F. (2009) 'Rassf family of tumor suppressor polypeptides', *The Journal of biological chemistry* 284(17): 11001-5.

Bachmann, I. M., Halvorsen, O. J., Collett, K., Stefansson, I. M., Straume, O., Haukaas, S. A., Salvesen, H. B., Otte, A. P. and Akslen, L. A. (2006) 'EZH2 expression is associated with high proliferation rate and aggressive tumor subgroups in cutaneous melanoma and cancers of the endometrium, prostate, and breast', *Journal of clinical oncology : official journal of the American Society of Clinical Oncology* 24(2): 268-73.

Bahrami, A., Ro, J. Y. and Ayala, A. G. (2007) 'An overview of testicular germ cell tumors', *Archives of pathology & laboratory medicine* 131(8): 1267-80.

Baumann, S., Keller, G., Puhringer, F., Napieralski, R., Feith, M., Langer, R., Hofler, H., Stein, H. J. and Sarbia, M. (2006) 'The prognostic impact of O6-Methylguanine-DNA Methyltransferase (MGMT) promotor hypermethylation in esophageal adenocarcinoma', *International journal of cancer. Journal international du cancer* 119(2): 264-8.

Bestor, T., Laudano, A., Mattaliano, R. and Ingram, V. (1988) 'Cloning and sequencing of a cDNA encoding DNA methyltransferase of mouse cells. The carboxyl-terminal domain of the mammalian enzymes is related to bacterial restriction methyltransferases', *Journal of molecular biology* 203(4): 971-83.

Beyrouthy, M. J., Garner, K. M., Hever, M. P., Freemantle, S. J., Eastman, A., Dmitrovsky, E. and Spinella, M. J. (2009) 'High DNA methyltransferase 3B expression mediates 5-aza-deoxycytidine hypersensitivity in testicular germ cell tumors', *Cancer research* 69(24): 9360-6.

Bianco, T., Chenevix-Trench, G., Walsh, D. C., Cooper, J. E. and Dobrovic, A. (2000) 'Tumour-specific distribution of BRCA1 promoter region methylation supports a pathogenetic role in breast and ovarian cancer', *Carcinogenesis* 21(2): 147-51.

Biermann, K., Heukamp, L. C., Steger, K., Zhou, H., Franke, F. E., Sonnack, V., Brehm, R., Berg, J., Bastian, P. J., Muller, S. C. et al. (2007) 'Genome-wide expression profiling reveals new insights into pathogenesis and progression of testicular germ cell tumors', *Cancer genomics & proteomics* 4(5): 359-67.

Biermann, K. and Steger, K. (2007) 'Epigenetics in male germ cells', *Journal of andrology* 28(4): 466-80.

Bracken, A. P., Pasini, D., Capra, M., Prosperini, E., Colli, E. and Helin, K. (2003) 'EZH2 is downstream of the pRB-E2F pathway, essential for proliferation and amplified in cancer', *The EMBO journal* 22(20): 5323-35.

Bratthauer, G. L. and Fanning, T. G. (1992) 'Active LINE-1 retrotransposons in human testicular cancer', *Oncogene* 7(3): 507-10.

Buermeyer, A. B., Wilson-Van Patten, C., Baker, S. M. and Liskay, R. M. (1999) 'The human MLH1 cDNA complements DNA mismatch repair defects in Mlh1-deficient mouse embryonic fibroblasts', *Cancer research* 59(3): 538-41.

Cabello, M. J., Grau, L., Franco, N., Orenes, E., Alvarez, M., Blanca, A., Heredero, O., Palacios, A., Urrutia, M., Fernandez, J. M. et al. (2011) 'Multiplexed methylation profiles of tumor suppressor genes in bladder cancer', *The Journal of molecular diagnostics : JMD* 13(1): 29-40.

Cao, R. and Zhang, Y. (2004) 'The functions of E(Z)/EZH2-mediated methylation of lysine 27 in histone H3', *Current opinion in genetics & development* 14(2): 155-64.

Cao, V. T., Jung, T. Y., Jung, S., Jin, S. G., Moon, K. S., Kim, I. Y., Kang, S. S., Park, C. S., Lee, K. H. and Chae, H. J. (2009) 'The correlation and prognostic significance of MGMT promoter methylation and MGMT protein in glioblastomas', *Neurosurgery* 65(5): 866-75; discussion 875.

Cecchi, C. (2002) 'Emx2: a gene responsible for cortical development, regionalization and area specification', *Gene* 291(1-2): 1-9.

Chaubert, P., Guillou, L., Kurt, A. M., Bertholet, M. M., Metthez, G., Leisinger, H. J., Bosman, F. and Shaw, P. (1997) 'Frequent p16INK4 (MTS1) gene inactivation in testicular germ cell tumors', *The American journal of pathology* 151(3): 859-65.

Chen, W. Y., Wang, D. H., Yen, R. C., Luo, J., Gu, W. and Baylin, S. B. (2005) 'Tumor suppressor HIC1 directly regulates SIRT1 to modulate p53-dependent DNA-damage responses', *Cell* 123(3): 437-48.

Chow, L. W., Zhu, L., Loo, W. T. and Lui, E. L. (2005) 'Aberrant methylation of cyclooxygenase-2 in breast cancer patients', *Biomedicine & pharmacotherapy = Biomedecine & pharmacotherapie* 59 Suppl 2: S264-7.

de Ruijter, A. J., van Gennip, A. H., Caron, H. N., Kemp, S. and van Kuilenburg, A. B. (2003) 'Histone deacetylases (HDACs): characterization of the classical HDAC family', *The Biochemical journal* 370(Pt 3): 737-49.

de Vries, A. and van Steeg, H. (1996) 'Xpa knockout mice', *Seminars in cancer biology* 7(5): 229-40.

Deng, C. X. and Brodie, S. G. (2000) 'Roles of BRCA1 and its interacting proteins', *BioEssays : news and reviews in molecular, cellular and developmental biology* 22(8): 728-37.

Dolle, P. (2009) 'Developmental expression of retinoic acid receptors (RARs)', *Nuclear receptor signaling* 7: e006.

Dong, S. M., Kim, H. S., Rha, S. H. and Sidransky, D. (2001) 'Promoter hypermethylation of multiple genes in carcinoma of the uterine cervix', *Clinical cancer research : an official journal of the American Association for Cancer Research* 7(7): 1982-6.

Dunn, B. K. (2003) 'Hypomethylation: one side of a larger picture', *Annals of the New York Academy of Sciences* 983: 28-42.

Dunwell, T. L., Hesson, L. B., Pavlova, T., Zabarovska, V., Kashuba, V., Catchpoole, D., Chiaramonte, R., Brini, A. T., Griffiths, M., Maher, E. R. et al. (2009) 'Epigenetic analysis of childhood acute lymphoblastic leukemia', *Epigenetics : official journal of the DNA Methylation Society* 4(3): 185-93.

Eckert, D., Biermann, K., Nettersheim, D., Gillis, A. J., Steger, K., Jack, H. M., Muller, A. M., Looijenga, L. H. and Schorle, H. (2008) 'Expression of BLIMP1/PRMT5 and concurrent histone H2A/H4 arginine 3 dimethylation in fetal germ cells, CIS/IGCNU and germ cell tumors', *BMC developmental biology* 8: 106.

Eden, A., Gaudet, F., Waghmare, A. and Jaenisch, R. (2003) 'Chromosomal instability and tumors promoted by DNA hypomethylation', *Science* 300(5618): 455.

Ehrlich, M. and Wang, R. Y. (1981) '5-Methylcytosine in eukaryotic DNA', *Science* 212(4501): 1350-7.

Ellinger, J., Albers, P., Perabo, F. G., Muller, S. C., von Ruecker, A. and Bastian, P. J. (2009) 'CpG island hypermethylation of cell-free circulating serum DNA in patients with testicular cancer', *The Journal of urology* 182(1): 324-9.

Estecio, M. R. and Issa, J. P. (2011) 'Dissecting DNA hypermethylation in cancer', *FEBS letters* 585(13): 2078-86.

Esteller, M. (2008) 'Epigenetics in cancer', *The New England journal of medicine* 358(11): 1148-59.

Esteller, M., Corn, P. G., Baylin, S. B. and Herman, J. G. (2001) 'A gene hypermethylation profile of human cancer', *Cancer research* 61(8): 3225-9.

Esteller, M., Levine, R., Baylin, S. B., Ellenson, L. H. and Herman, J. G. (1998) 'MLH1 promoter hypermethylation is associated with the microsatellite instability phenotype in sporadic endometrial carcinomas', *Oncogene* 17(18): 2413-7.

Fackler, M. J., McVeigh, M., Evron, E., Garrett, E., Mehrotra, J., Polyak, K., Sukumar, S. and Argani, P. (2003) 'DNA methylation of RASSF1A, HIN-1, RAR-beta, Cyclin D2 and Twist in in situ and invasive lobular breast carcinoma', *International journal of cancer. Journal international du cancer* 107(6): 970-5.

Faure, A. K., Pivot-Pajot, C., Kerjean, A., Hazzouri, M., Pelletier, R., Peoc'h, M., Sele, B., Khochbin, S. and Rousseaux, S. (2003) 'Misregulation of histone acetylation in Sertoli cell-only syndrome and testicular cancer', *Molecular human reproduction* 9(12): 757-63.

Feng, Q., Hawes, S. E., Stern, J. E., Wiens, L., Lu, H., Dong, Z. M., Jordan, C. D., Kiviat, N. B. and Vesselle, H. (2008) 'DNA methylation in tumor and matched normal tissues from non-small cell lung cancer patients', *Cancer epidemiology, biomarkers & prevention : a publication of the American Association for Cancer Research, cosponsored by the American Society of Preventive Oncology* 17(3): 645-54.

Feng, Q., Stern, J. E., Hawes, S. E., Lu, H., Jiang, M. and Kiviat, N. B. (2010) 'DNA methylation changes in normal liver tissues and hepatocellular carcinoma with different viral infection', *Experimental and molecular pathology* 88(2): 287-92.

Fu, M., Lui, V. C., Sham, M. H., Cheung, A. N. and Tam, P. K. (2003) 'HOXB5 expression is spatially and temporarily regulated in human embryonic gut during neural crest cell colonization and differentiation of enteric neuroblasts', *Developmental dynamics : an official publication of the American Association of Anatomists* 228(1): 1-10.

Fujii, H., Biel, M. A., Zhou, W., Weitzman, S. A., Baylin, S. B. and Gabrielson, E. (1998) 'Methylation of the HIC-1 candidate tumor suppressor gene in human breast cancer', *Oncogene* 16(16): 2159-64.

Gama-Sosa, M. A., Slagel, V. A., Trewyn, R. W., Oxenhandler, R., Kuo, K. C., Gehrke, C. W. and Ehrlich, M. (1983) 'The 5-methylcytosine content of DNA from human tumors', *Nucleic acids research* 11(19): 6883-94.

Gaskell, T. L., Esnal, A., Robinson, L. L., Anderson, R. A. and Saunders, P. T. (2004) 'Immunohistochemical profiling of germ cells within the human fetal testis: identification of three subpopulations', *Biology of reproduction* 71(6): 2012-21.

Gjerset, R. A. (2006) 'DNA damage, p14ARF, nucleophosmin (NPM/B23), and cancer', *Journal of molecular histology* 37(5-7): 239-51.

Godmann, M., Lambrot, R. and Kimmins, S. (2009) 'The dynamic epigenetic program in male germ cells: Its role in spermatogenesis, testis cancer, and its response to the environment', *Microscopy research and technique* 72(8): 603-19.

Goel, A., Arnold, C. N., Tassone, P., Chang, D. K., Niedzwiecki, D., Dowell, J. M., Wasserman, L., Compton, C., Mayer, R. J., Bertagnolli, M. M. et al. (2004) 'Epigenetic inactivation of RUNX3 in microsatellite unstable sporadic colon cancers', *International journal of cancer. Journal international du cancer* 112(5): 754-9.

Gong, Y., Guo, M. Z., Ye, Z. J., Zhang, X. L., Zhao, Y. L. and Yang, Y. S. (2011) 'Silence of HIN-1 expression through methylation of its gene promoter in gastric cancer', *World journal of gastroenterology : WJG* 17(4): 526-33.

Gordon, M. and Baksh, S. (2011) 'RASSF1A: Not a prototypical Ras effector', *Small GTPases* 2(3): 148-157.

Guerrero-Preston, R., Soudry, E., Acero, J., Orera, M., Moreno-Lopez, L., Macia-Colon, G., Jaffe, A., Berdasco, M., Ili-Gangas, C., Brebi-Mieville, P. et al. (2011) 'NID2 and HOXA9 promoter hypermethylation as biomarkers for prevention and early detection in oral cavity squamous cell carcinoma tissues and saliva', *Cancer prevention research* 4(7): 1061-72.

Hamilton, G., Yee, K. S., Scrace, S. and O'Neill, E. (2009) 'ATM regulates a RASSF1A-dependent DNA damage response', *Current biology : CB* 19(23): 2020-5.

Hatziapostolou, M. and Iliopoulos, D. (2011) 'Epigenetic aberrations during oncogenesis', *Cellular and molecular life sciences : CMLS* 68(10): 1681-702.

Hayashi, K., Yoshida, K. and Matsui, Y. (2005) 'A histone H3 methyltransferase controls epigenetic events required for meiotic prophase', *Nature* 438(7066): 374-8.

Herman, J. G., Umar, A., Polyak, K., Graff, J. R., Ahuja, N., Issa, J. P., Markowitz, S., Willson, J. K., Hamilton, S. R., Kinzler, K. W. et al. (1998) 'Incidence and functional consequences of hMLH1 promoter hypermethylation in colorectal carcinoma', *Proceedings of the National Academy of Sciences of the United States of America* 95(12): 6870-5.

Hiltunen, M. O., Alhonen, L., Koistinaho, J., Myohanen, S., Paakkonen, M., Marin, S., Kosma, V. M. and Janne, J. (1997) 'Hypermethylation of the APC (adenomatous polyposis coli) gene promoter region in human colorectal carcinoma', *International journal of cancer. Journal international du cancer* 70(6): 644-8.

Hinz, S., Magheli, A., Weikert, S., Schulze, W., Krause, H., Schrader, M., Miller, K. and Kempkensteffen, C. (2010) 'Deregulation of EZH2 expression in human spermatogenic disorders and testicular germ cell tumors', *World journal of urology* 28(5): 631-5.

Hirohashi, S. (1998) 'Inactivation of the E-cadherin-mediated cell adhesion system in human cancers', *The American journal of pathology* 153(2): 333-9.

Honorio, S., Agathanggelou, A., Wernert, N., Rothe, M., Maher, E. R. and Latif, F. (2003) 'Frequent epigenetic inactivation of the RASSF1A tumour suppressor gene in testicular tumours and distinct methylation profiles of seminoma and nonseminoma testicular germ cell tumours', *Oncogene* 22(3): 461-6.

Hsu, H. S., Chen, T. P., Hung, C. H., Wen, C. K., Lin, R. K., Lee, H. C. and Wang, Y. C. (2007) 'Characterization of a multiple epigenetic marker panel for lung cancer detection and risk assessment in plasma', *Cancer* 110(9): 2019-26.

Huddart, R. A., Wooster, R., Horwich, A. and Cooper, C. S. (1995) 'Microsatellite instability in human testicular germ cell tumours', *British journal of cancer* 72(3): 642-5.

Hwang, K. T., Han, W., Bae, J. Y., Hwang, S. E., Shin, H. J., Lee, J. E., Kim, S. W., Min, H. J. and Noh, D. Y. (2007) 'Downregulation of the RUNX3 gene by promoter hypermethylation and hemizygous deletion in breast cancer', *Journal of Korean medical science* 22 Suppl: S24-31.

Hwang, S. H., Kim, K. U., Kim, J. E., Kim, H. H., Lee, M. K., Lee, C. H., Lee, S. Y., Oh, T. and An, S. (2011) 'Detection of HOXA9 gene methylation in tumor tissues and induced sputum samples from primary lung cancer patients', *Clinical chemistry and laboratory medicine : CCLM / FESCC* 49(4): 699-704.

Ishii, T., Kohu, K., Yamada, S., Ishidoya, S., Kanto, S., Fuji, H., Moriya, T., Satake, M. and Arai, Y. (2007) 'Up-regulation of DNA-methyltransferase 3A expression is associated with hypomethylation of intron 25 in human testicular germ cell tumors', *The Tohoku journal of experimental medicine* 212(2): 177-90.

Iyer, P., Zekri, A. R., Hung, C. W., Schiefelbein, E., Ismail, K., Hablas, A., Seifeldin, I. A. and Soliman, A. S. (2010) 'Concordance of DNA methylation pattern in plasma and tumor DNA of Egyptian hepatocellular carcinoma patients', *Experimental and molecular pathology* 88(1): 107-11.

Jing, S., Wen, D., Yu, Y., Holst, P. L., Luo, Y., Fang, M., Tamir, R., Antonio, L., Hu, Z., Cupples, R. et al. (1996) 'GDNF-induced activation of the ret protein tyrosine kinase is mediated by GDNFR-alpha, a novel receptor for GDNF', *Cell* 85(7): 1113-24.

Jurkowska, R. Z., Jurkowski, T. P. and Jeltsch, A. (2011) 'Structure and function of mammalian DNA methyltransferases', *Chembiochem : a European journal of chemical biology* 12(2): 206-22.

Kaneda, M., Okano, M., Hata, K., Sado, T., Tsujimoto, N., Li, E. and Sasaki, H. (2004) 'Essential role for de novo DNA methyltransferase Dnmt3a in paternal and maternal imprinting', *Nature* 429(6994): 900-3.

Kato, N., Tamura, G., Fukase, M., Shibuya, H. and Motoyama, T. (2003) 'Hypermethylation of the RUNX3 gene promoter in testicular yolk sac tumor of infants', *The American journal of pathology* 163(2): 387-91.

Kawakami, K., Brabender, J., Lord, R. V., Groshen, S., Greenwald, B. D., Krasna, M. J., Yin, J., Fleisher, A. S., Abraham, J. M., Beer, D. G. et al. (2000) 'Hypermethylated APC DNA in plasma and prognosis of patients with esophageal adenocarcinoma', *Journal of the National Cancer Institute* 92(22): 1805-11.

Kawakami, T., Okamoto, K., Kataoka, A., Koizumi, S., Iwaki, H., Sugihara, H., Reeve, A. E., Ogawa, O. and Okada, Y. (2003) 'Multipoint methylation analysis indicates a distinctive epigenetic phenotype among testicular germ cell tumors and testicular malignant lymphomas', *Genes, chromosomes & cancer* 38(1): 97-101.

Kempkensteffen, C., Christoph, F., Weikert, S., Krause, H., Kollermann, J., Schostak, M., Miller, K. and Schrader, M. (2006) 'Epigenetic silencing of the putative tumor suppressor gene testisin in testicular germ cell tumors', *Journal of cancer research and clinical oncology* 132(12): 765-70.

Ki, K. D., Lee, S. K., Tong, S. Y., Lee, J. M., Song, D. H. and Chi, S. G. (2008) 'Role of 5'-CpG island hypermethylation of the FHIT gene in cervical carcinoma', *Journal of gynecologic oncology* 19(2): 117-22.

Kim, W. J., Kim, E. J., Jeong, P., Quan, C., Kim, J., Li, Q. L., Yang, J. O., Ito, Y. and Bae, S. C. (2005) 'RUNX3 inactivation by point mutations and aberrant DNA methylation in bladder tumors', *Cancer research* 65(20): 9347-54.

Korkola, J. E., Houldsworth, J., Dobrzynski, D., Olshen, A. B., Reuter, V. E., Bosl, G. J. and Chaganti, R. S. (2005) 'Gene expression-based classification of nonseminomatous male germ cell tumors', *Oncogene* 24(32): 5101-7.

Koul, S., Houldsworth, J., Mansukhani, M. M., Donadio, A., McKiernan, J. M., Reuter, V. E., Bosl, G. J., Chaganti, R. S. and Murty, V. V. (2002) 'Characteristic promoter hypermethylation signatures in male germ cell tumors', *Molecular cancer* 1: 8.

Koul, S., McKiernan, J. M., Narayan, G., Houldsworth, J., Bacik, J., Dobrzynski, D. L., Assaad, A. M., Mansukhani, M., Reuter, V. E., Bosl, G. J. et al. (2004) 'Role of promoter hypermethylation in Cisplatin treatment response of male germ cell tumors', *Molecular cancer* 3: 16.

Krop, I., Player, A., Tablante, A., Taylor-Parker, M., Lahti-Domenici, J., Fukuoka, J., Batra, S. K., Papadopoulos, N., Richards, W. G., Sugarbaker, D. J. et al. (2004) 'Frequent HIN-1 promoter methylation and lack of expression in multiple human tumor types', *Molecular cancer research : MCR* 2(9): 489-94.

Kuroki, T., Trapasso, F., Yendamuri, S., Matsuyama, A., Alder, H., Mori, M. and Croce, C. M. (2003) 'Promoter hypermethylation of RASSF1A in esophageal squamous cell carcinoma', *Clinical cancer research : an official journal of the American Association for Cancer Research* 9(4): 1441-5.

Lawrence, H. J., Helgason, C. D., Sauvageau, G., Fong, S., Izon, D. J., Humphries, R. K. and Largman, C. (1997) 'Mice bearing a targeted interruption of the homeobox gene HOXA9 have defects in myeloid, erythroid, and lymphoid hematopoiesis', *Blood* 89(6): 1922-30.

Leung, S. Y., Yuen, S. T., Chung, L. P., Chu, K. M., Chan, A. S. and Ho, J. C. (1999) 'hMLH1 promoter methylation and lack of hMLH1 expression in sporadic gastric carcinomas with high-frequency microsatellite instability', *Cancer research* 59(1): 159-64.

Leveille, F., Blom, E., Medhurst, A. L., Bier, P., Laghmani el, H., Johnson, M., Rooimans, M. A., Sobeck, A., Waisfisz, Q., Arwert, F. et al. (2004) 'The Fanconi anemia gene product FANCF is a flexible adaptor protein', *The Journal of biological chemistry* 279(38): 39421-30.

Li, Q. L., Kim, H. R., Kim, W. J., Choi, J. K., Lee, Y. H., Kim, H. M., Li, L. S., Kim, H., Chang, J., Ito, Y. et al. (2004) 'Transcriptional silencing of the RUNX3 gene by CpG hypermethylation is associated with lung cancer', *Biochemical and biophysical research communications* 314(1): 223-8.

Lin, W. H., Huang, C. J., Liu, M. W., Chang, H. M., Chen, Y. J., Tai, T. Y. and Chuang, L. M. (2001) 'Cloning, mapping, and characterization of the human sorbin and SH3 domain containing 1 (SORBS1) gene: a protein associated with c-Abl during insulin signaling in the hepatoma cell line Hep3B', *Genomics* 74(1): 12-20.

Lind, G. E., Skotheim, R. I., Fraga, M. F., Abeler, V. M., Esteller, M. and Lothe, R. A. (2006) 'Novel epigenetically deregulated genes in testicular cancer include homeobox genes and SCGB3A1 (HIN-1)', *The Journal of pathology* 210(4): 441-9.

Lind, G. E., Skotheim, R. I. and Lothe, R. A. (2007) 'The epigenome of testicular germ cell tumors', *APMIS : acta pathologica, microbiologica, et immunologica Scandinavica* 115(10): 1147-60.

Lusher, M. E., Lindsey, J. C., Latif, F., Pearson, A. D., Ellison, D. W. and Clifford, S. C. (2002) 'Biallelic epigenetic inactivation of the RASSF1A tumor suppressor gene in medulloblastoma development', *Cancer research* 62(20): 5906-11.

Maekawa, M. and Watanabe, Y. (2007) 'Epigenetics: relations to disease and laboratory findings', *Current medicinal chemistry* 14(25): 2642-53.

Manton, K. J., Douglas, M. L., Netzel-Arnett, S., Fitzpatrick, D. R., Nicol, D. L., Boyd, A. W., Clements, J. A. and Antalis, T. M. (2005) 'Hypermethylation of the 5' CpG island of the gene encoding the serine protease Testisin promotes its loss in testicular tumorigenesis', *British journal of cancer* 92(4): 760-9.

Maruyama, R., Toyooka, S., Toyooka, K. O., Harada, K., Virmani, A. K., Zochbauer-Muller, S., Farinas, A. J., Vakar-Lopez, F., Minna, J. D., Sagalowsky, A. et al. (2001) 'Aberrant promoter methylation profile of bladder cancer and its relationship to clinicopathological features', *Cancer research* 61(24): 8659-63.

Meng, X., Lindahl, M., Hyvonen, M. E., Parvinen, M., de Rooij, D. G., Hess, M. W., Raatikainen-Ahokas, A., Sainio, K., Rauvala, H., Lakso, M. et al. (2000) 'Regulation of cell fate decision of undifferentiated spermatogonia by GDNF', *Science* 287(5457): 1489-93.

Mitra, S. (2007) 'MGMT: a personal perspective', *DNA repair* 6(8): 1064-70.

Muller-Thomas, C., Schuster, T., Peschel, C. and Gotze, K. S. (2009) 'A limited number of 5-azacitidine cycles can be effective treatment in MDS', *Annals of hematology* 88(3): 213-9.

Murata, H., Khattar, N. H., Kang, Y., Gu, L. and Li, G. M. (2002) 'Genetic and epigenetic modification of mismatch repair genes hMSH2 and hMLH1 in sporadic breast cancer with microsatellite instability', *Oncogene* 21(37): 5696-703.

Narayan, A., Ji, W., Zhang, X. Y., Marrogi, A., Graff, J. R., Baylin, S. B. and Ehrlich, M. (1998) 'Hypomethylation of pericentromeric DNA in breast adenocarcinomas', *International journal of cancer. Journal international du cancer* 77(6): 833-8.

Narayan, G., Arias-Pulido, H., Koul, S., Vargas, H., Zhang, F. F., Villella, J., Schneider, A., Terry, M. B., Mansukhani, M. and Murty, V. V. (2003) 'Frequent promoter methylation of CDH1, DAPK, RARB, and HIC1 genes in carcinoma of cervix uteri: its relationship to clinical outcome', *Molecular cancer* 2: 24.

Narayan, G., Arias-Pulido, H., Nandula, S. V., Basso, K., Sugirtharaj, D. D., Vargas, H., Mansukhani, M., Villella, J., Meyer, L., Schneider, A. et al. (2004) 'Promoter hypermethylation of FANCF: disruption of Fanconi Anemia-BRCA pathway in cervical cancer', *Cancer research* 64(9): 2994-7.

Nettersheim, D., Biermann, K., Gillis, A. J., Steger, K., Looijenga, L. H. and Schorle, H. (2011) 'NANOG promoter methylation and expression correlation during normal and malignant human germ cell development', *Epigenetics : official journal of the DNA Methylation Society* 6(1): 114-22.

Okamoto, J., Hirata, T., Chen, Z., Zhou, H. M., Mikami, I., Li, H., Yagui-Beltran, A., Johansson, M., Coussens, L. M., Clement, G. et al. (2010) 'EMX2 is epigenetically silenced and suppresses growth in human lung cancer', *Oncogene* 29(44): 5969-75.

Okano, M., Bell, D. W., Haber, D. A. and Li, E. (1999) 'DNA methyltransferases Dnmt3a and Dnmt3b are essential for de novo methylation and mammalian development', *Cell* 99(3): 247-57.

Olasz, J., Mandoky, L., Geczi, L., Bodrogi, I., Csuka, O. and Bak, M. (2005) 'Influence of hMLH1 methylation, mismatch repair deficiency and microsatellite instability on chemoresistance of testicular germ-cell tumors', *Anticancer research* 25(6B): 4319-24.

Omisanjo, O. A., Biermann, K., Hartmann, S., Heukamp, L. C., Sonnack, V., Hild, A., Brehm, R., Bergmann, M., Weidner, W. and Steger, K. (2007) 'DNMT1 and HDAC1 gene expression in impaired spermatogenesis and testicular cancer', *Histochemistry and cell biology* 127(2): 175-81.

Otto, F., Lubbert, M. and Stock, M. (2003) 'Upstream and downstream targets of RUNX proteins', *Journal of cellular biochemistry* 89(1): 9-18.

Payne, C. and Braun, R. E. (2006) 'Histone lysine trimethylation exhibits a distinct perinuclear distribution in Plzf-expressing spermatogonia', *Developmental biology* 293(2): 461-72.

Payne, C. J., Gallagher, S. J., Foreman, O., Dannenberg, J. H., Depinho, R. A. and Braun, R. E. (2010) 'Sin3a is required by sertoli cells to establish a niche for undifferentiated spermatogonia, germ cell tumors, and spermatid elongation', *Stem Cells* 28(8): 1424-34.

Peters, A. H., O'Carroll, D., Scherthan, H., Mechtler, K., Sauer, S., Schofer, C., Weipoltshammer, K., Pagani, M., Lachner, M., Kohlmaier, A. et al. (2001) 'Loss of the Suv39h histone methyltransferases impairs mammalian heterochromatin and genome stability', *Cell* 107(3): 323-37.

Pfeifer, G. P., Yoon, J. H., Liu, L., Tommasi, S., Wilczynski, S. P. and Dammann, R. (2002) 'Methylation of the RASSF1A gene in human cancers', *Biological chemistry* 383(6): 907-14.

Postel, E. H., Berberich, S. J., Rooney, J. W. and Kaetzel, D. M. (2000) 'Human NM23/nucleoside diphosphate kinase regulates gene expression through DNA binding to nuclease-hypersensitive transcriptional elements', *Journal of bioenergetics and biomembranes* 32(3): 277-84.

Qu, G., Dubeau, L., Narayan, A., Yu, M. C. and Ehrlich, M. (1999) 'Satellite DNA hypomethylation vs. overall genomic hypomethylation in ovarian epithelial tumors of different malignant potential', *Mutation research* 423(1-2): 91-101.

Rawlings, N. D. and Barrett, A. J. (1994) 'Families of serine peptidases', *Methods in enzymology* 244: 19-61.

Rice, J. C., Ozcelik, H., Maxeiner, P., Andrulis, I. and Futscher, B. W. (2000) 'Methylation of the BRCA1 promoter is associated with decreased BRCA1 mRNA levels in clinical breast cancer specimens', *Carcinogenesis* 21(9): 1761-5.

Rizzo, M. T. (2011) 'Cyclooxygenase-2 in oncogenesis', *Clinica chimica acta; international journal of clinical chemistry* 412(9-10): 671-87.

Rodriguez, J., Frigola, J., Vendrell, E., Risques, R. A., Fraga, M. F., Morales, C., Moreno, V., Esteller, M., Capella, G., Ribas, M. et al. (2006) 'Chromosomal instability correlates with genome-wide DNA demethylation in human primary colorectal cancers', *Cancer research* 66(17): 8462-9468.

Roman-Gomez, J., Castillejo, J. A., Jimenez, A., Cervantes, F., Boque, C., Hermosin, L., Leon, A., Granena, A., Colomer, D., Heiniger, A. et al. (2003) 'Cadherin-13, a mediator of calcium-dependent cell-cell adhesion, is silenced by methylation in chronic myeloid leukemia and correlates with pretreatment risk profile and cytogenetic response to interferon alfa', *Journal of clinical oncology : official journal of the American Society of Clinical Oncology* 21(8): 1472-9.

Sakai, T., Toguchida, J., Ohtani, N., Yandell, D. W., Rapaport, J. M. and Dryja, T. P. (1991) 'Allele-specific hypermethylation of the retinoblastoma tumor-suppressor gene', *American journal of human genetics* 48(5): 880-8.

Saldivar, J. C., Shibata, H. and Huebner, K. (2010) 'Pathology and biology associated with the fragile FHIT gene and gene product', *Journal of cellular biochemistry* 109(5): 858-65.

Senda, T., Iizuka-Kogo, A., Onouchi, T. and Shimomura, A. (2007) 'Adenomatous polyposis coli (APC) plays multiple roles in the intestinal and colorectal epithelia', *Medical molecular morphology* 40(2): 68-81.

Sette, C., Dolci, S., Geremia, R. and Rossi, P. (2000) 'The role of stem cell factor and of alternative c-kit gene products in the establishment, maintenance and function of germ cells', *The International journal of developmental biology* 44(6): 599-608.

Shames, D. S., Girard, L., Gao, B., Sato, M., Lewis, C. M., Shivapurkar, N., Jiang, A., Perou, C. M., Kim, Y. H., Pollack, J. R. et al. (2006) 'A genome-wide screen for promoter methylation in lung cancer identifies novel methylation markers for multiple malignancies', *PLoS medicine* 3(12): e486.

Singal, R., Ferdinand, L., Reis, I. M. and Schlesselman, J. J. (2004) 'Methylation of multiple genes in prostate cancer and the relationship with clinicopathological features of disease', *Oncology reports* 12(3): 631-7.

Skotheim, R. I., Lind, G. E., Monni, O., Nesland, J. M., Abeler, V. M., Fossa, S. D., Duale, N., Brunborg, G., Kallioniemi, O., Andrews, P. W. et al. (2005) 'Differentiation of human embryonal carcinomas in vitro and in vivo reveals expression profiles relevant to normal development', *Cancer research* 65(13): 5588-98.

Smith-Sorensen, B., Lind, G. E., Skotheim, R. I., Fossa, S. D., Fodstad, O., Stenwig, A. E., Jakobsen, K. S. and Lothe, R. A. (2002) 'Frequent promoter hypermethylation of the O6-Methylguanine-DNA Methyltransferase (MGMT) gene in testicular cancer', *Oncogene* 21(57): 8878-84.

Spugnardi, M., Tommasi, S., Dammann, R., Pfeifer, G. P. and Hoon, D. S. (2003) 'Epigenetic inactivation of RAS association domain family protein 1 (RASSF1A) in malignant cutaneous melanoma', *Cancer research* 63(7): 1639-43.

Strange, R. C., Spiteri, M. A., Ramachandran, S. and Fryer, A. A. (2001) 'Glutathione-S-transferase family of enzymes', *Mutation research* 482(1-2): 21-6.

Strathdee, G., MacKean, M. J., Illand, M. and Brown, R. (1999) 'A role for methylation of the hMLH1 promoter in loss of hMLH1 expression and drug resistance in ovarian cancer', *Oncogene* 18(14): 2335-41.

Suzuki, A., Raya, A., Kawakami, Y., Morita, M., Matsui, T., Nakashima, K., Gage, F. H., Rodriguez-Esteban, C. and Izpisua Belmonte, J. C. (2006) 'Nanog binds to Smad1 and blocks bone morphogenetic protein-induced differentiation of embryonic stem cells', *Proceedings of the National Academy of Sciences of the United States of America* 103(27): 10294-9.

Suzuki, M. M. and Bird, A. (2008) 'DNA methylation landscapes: provocative insights from epigenomics', *Nature reviews. Genetics* 9(6): 465-76.

Tachibana, M., Nozaki, M., Takeda, N. and Shinkai, Y. (2007) 'Functional dynamics of H3K9 methylation during meiotic prophase progression', *The EMBO journal* 26(14): 3346-59.

Tajima, Y., Sawada, K., Morimoto, T. and Nishimune, Y. (1994) 'Switching of mouse spermatogonial proliferation from the c-kit receptor-independent type to the receptor-dependent type during differentiation', *Journal of reproduction and fertility* 102(1): 117-22.

Taniguchi, T., Tischkowitz, M., Ameziane, N., Hodgson, S. V., Mathew, C. G., Joenje, H., Mok, S. C. and D'Andrea, A. D. (2003) 'Disruption of the Fanconi anemia-BRCA pathway in cisplatin-sensitive ovarian tumors', *Nature medicine* 9(5): 568-74.

Tian, Y., Hou, Y., Zhou, X., Cheng, H. and Zhou, R. (2011) 'Tumor suppressor RASSF1A promoter: p53 binding and methylation', *PloS one* 6(2): e17017.

Tomita, T. and Kimura, S. (2008) 'Regulation of mouse Scgb3a1 gene expression by NF-Y and association of CpG methylation with its tissue-specific expression', *BMC molecular biology* 9: 5.

Toyooka, K. O., Toyooka, S., Virmani, A. K., Sathyanarayana, U. G., Euhus, D. M., Gilcrease, M., Minna, J. D. and Gazdar, A. F. (2001) 'Loss of expression and aberrant methylation of the CDH13 (H-cadherin) gene in breast and lung carcinomas', *Cancer research* 61(11): 4556-60.

Troy, P. J., Daftary, G. S., Bagot, C. N. and Taylor, H. S. (2003) 'Transcriptional repression of peri-implantation EMX2 expression in mammalian reproduction by HOXA10', *Molecular and cellular biology* 23(1): 1-13.

Uhlmann, K., Rohde, K., Zeller, C., Szymas, J., Vogel, S., Marczinek, K., Thiel, G., Nurnberg, P. and Laird, P. W. (2003) 'Distinct methylation profiles of glioma subtypes', *International journal of cancer. Journal international du cancer* 106(1): 52-9.

Ushida, H., Kawakami, T., Minami, K., Chano, T., Okabe, H., Okada, Y. and Okamoto, K. (2011) 'Methylation profile of DNA repetitive elements in human testicular germ cell tumor', *Molecular carcinogenesis*.

Varambally, S., Dhanasekaran, S. M., Zhou, M., Barrette, T. R., Kumar-Sinha, C., Sanda, M. G., Ghosh, D., Pienta, K. J., Sewalt, R. G., Otte, A. P. et al. (2002) 'The polycomb group protein EZH2 is involved in progression of prostate cancer', *Nature* 419(6907): 624-9.

Viglietto, G., Dolci, S., Bruni, P., Baldassarre, G., Chiariotti, L., Melillo, R. M., Salvatore, G., Chiappetta, G., Sferratore, F., Fusco, A. et al. (2000) 'Glial cell line-derived neutrotrophic factor and neurturin can act as paracrine growth factors stimulating DNA synthesis of Ret-expressing spermatogonia', *International journal of oncology* 16(4): 689-94.

Virmani, A. K., Rathi, A., Sathyanarayana, U. G., Padar, A., Huang, C. X., Cunnigham, H. T., Farinas, A. J., Milchgrub, S., Euhus, D. M., Gilcrease, M. et al. (2001) 'Aberrant methylation of the adenomatous polyposis coli (APC) gene promoter 1A in breast and lung carcinomas', *Clinical cancer research : an official journal of the American Association for Cancer Research* 7(7): 1998-2004.

Volpe, M. V., Martin, A., Vosatka, R. J., Mazzoni, C. L. and Nielsen, H. C. (1997) 'Hoxb-5 expression in the developing mouse lung suggests a role in branching morphogenesis and epithelial cell fate', *Histochemistry and cell biology* 108(6): 495-504.

Wali, A. (2010) 'FHIT: doubts are clear now', *TheScientificWorldJournal* 10: 1142-51.

Wang, Y., Zhang, D., Zheng, W., Luo, J., Bai, Y. and Lu, Z. (2008) 'Multiple gene methylation of nonsmall cell lung cancers evaluated with 3-dimensional microarray', *Cancer* 112(6): 1325-36.

Wermann, H., Stoop, H., Gillis, A. J., Honecker, F., van Gurp, R. J., Ammerpohl, O., Richter, J., Oosterhuis, J. W., Bokemeyer, C. and Looijenga, L. H. (2010) 'Global DNA methylation in fetal human germ cells and germ cell tumours: association with differentiation and cisplatin resistance', *The Journal of pathology* 221(4): 433-42.

Wolf, P., Hu, Y. C., Doffek, K., Sidransky, D. and Ahrendt, S. A. (2001) 'O(6)-Methylguanine-DNA methyltransferase promoter hypermethylation shifts the p53 mutational spectrum in non-small cell lung cancer', *Cancer research* 61(22): 8113-7.

Wong, T. S., Kwong, D. L., Sham, J. S., Tsao, S. W., Wei, W. I., Kwong, Y. L. and Yuen, A. P. (2003) 'Promoter hypermethylation of high-in-normal 1 gene in primary nasopharyngeal carcinoma', *Clinical cancer research : an official journal of the American Association for Cancer Research* 9(8): 3042-6.

Wu, Q., Lothe, R. A., Ahlquist, T., Silins, I., Trope, C. G., Micci, F., Nesland, J. M., Suo, Z. and Lind, G. E. (2007) 'DNA methylation profiling of ovarian carcinomas and their in vitro models identifies HOXA9, HOXB5, SCGB3A1, and CRABP1 as novel targets', *Molecular cancer* 6: 45.

Xiao, W. H. and Liu, W. W. (2004) 'Hemizygous deletion and hypermethylation of RUNX3 gene in hepatocellular carcinoma', *World journal of gastroenterology : WJG* 10(3): 376-80.

Yegnasubramanian, S., Kowalski, J., Gonzalgo, M. L., Zahurak, M., Piantadosi, S., Walsh, P. C., Bova, G. S., De Marzo, A. M., Isaacs, W. B. and Nelson, W. G. (2004) 'Hypermethylation of CpG islands in primary and metastatic human prostate cancer', *Cancer research* 64(6): 1975-86.

Yu, J., Leung, W. K., Lee, T. L., Tse, P. C., To, K. F. and Sung, J. J. (2003) 'Promoter hypermethylation of cyclooxygenase-2 in gastric carcinoma', *International journal of oncology* 22(5): 1025-31.

Yu, J., Mallon, M. A., Zhang, W., Freimuth, R. R., Marsh, S., Watson, M. A., Goodfellow, P. J. and McLeod, H. L. (2006) 'DNA repair pathway profiling and microsatellite instability in colorectal cancer', *Clinical cancer research : an official journal of the American Association for Cancer Research* 12(17): 5104-11.

Zhang, Y. J., Chen, Y., Ahsan, H., Lunn, R. M., Lee, P. H., Chen, C. J. and Santella, R. M. (2003) 'Inactivation of the DNA repair gene O6-methylguanine-DNA methyltransferase by promoter hypermethylation and its relationship to aflatoxin B1-DNA adducts and p53 mutation in hepatocellular carcinoma', *International journal of cancer. Journal international du cancer* 103(4): 440-4.

7

Claudins and Germ Cell Tumors

Ylermi Soini
Department of Pathology and Forensic Medicine, Institute of Clinical Medicine, Pathology and Forensic Medicine, School of Medicine, University of Eastern Finland, Cancer Center of Eastern Finland, Kuopio, Finland

1. Introduction

Tight junctions are cellular structures present in epithelial, endothelial and mesothelial cells (1, 2, 3). They are located at the apicolateral part of the cell membrane and regulate the paracellular permeability of cell layers which is called the gate function (4). They also have a fence function segregating the apical region of the cell membrane from the lateral parts preventing proteins of the apical area from mixing up with those of the lateral regions (1,4). Tight junctions also take part in determination of cellular polarity (1,4). They prevent pathogens from invading into the subepithelial tissues and thus can be considered to represent one part of the innate immune system (5).

In freeze fraction electron microscopy tight junctions form a beltlike branching structure around the cell which varies from 0.27µm to 0.37µm in thickness which depends on the cell type (6). Tight junctions are composed of membrane proteins and scaffolding proteins.The former include claudins, occludin, tricellulin and junctional adhesion molecules (7). Claudins, occluding and tricellulin have four transmembrane domains while junctional adhesion molecules have only one (7). Scaffolding proteins mediate interactions between tight junctions and the interior compartments of the cells. They include ZO-1 (Zona occludens-1), ZO-2, ZO-3, MAGI-1 (membrane-associated guanylate kinase with inverted orientation-1), cingulin and MUPP1 (multi-PDZ domain protein 1) (1,7).

2. Claudins

Claudins are tight junction proteins responsible for the regulation of paracellular permeability in cell layers. There are 27 claudins known and the diversity of claudins is the basis for differences in the solute and electrical permeability in different cell layers (1,8) (Table 1). In kidney tubules different claudins are expressed in different areas of the nephron determining the solute and electrolytic permeability in different regions of the kidney tubule (9). A similar segmental distribution in claudin expression is observed in the gut (10). Claudins do not share structural resemblance to either occludin or tricellulin (11).

Claudins are key components of tight junctions (1,4). They are 21-28kDa proteins containing an aminoterminal intracellular part, four transmembrane domains, two extracellular loops, an intracellular loop and an intracellular carboxyterminal end (1,4,5,7). The carboxyterminal

Claudin	Chromosomal location	Molecular weight (kDa)	Mutations/ disease	Splice variants	Other aspects
CLD1	3q28-29	22.7	Ictyosis, Sclerosing cholangitis		Entry cofactor for hepatitis C virus, right-left patterning in embryogenesis, knockdown causes transdermal water loss
CLD2	Xq22.3-q23	24.5	-	5	Knockdown prevents bile canalicular formation
CLD3	7q11.23	23.3			Receptor for CPE
CLD4	7q11.23	22.0			Receptor for CPE
CLD5	22q11.21	23.1			Present mainly in endothelium, heart development in Xenopus, knockdown causes disturbances in BBB function
CLD6	16p13.3	23.3			Entry cofactor for hepatitis C virus
CLD7	17	22.4		3	Knockdown decreases Cloride permeability
CLD8	21.22.11	24.8			
CLD9	16p13.3	22.8			Entry cofactor for hepatitis C virus
CLD10	13q31-34	24.2-24.5		6	
CLD11	3q26.2-q26.3	21.9	Deafness, Sertoli cell dysfunction		Knockdown causes nerve conduction disturbances, male sterility, deafness
CLD12	7q21	27.1		3	D vitamin induced Ca abrorption from enterocytes
CLD14	21q22.3	25.7	Sensoryneural deafness	5	Reduced mineral bone density, kidney stones, knockout causes deafness
CLD15	7q11.22	24.3		2	Megaintestine in knockout mice
CLD16	3q28	33.8	Hypomagnese mia type 3		
CLD17	21q22.11	24.6			Intronless gene
CLD18	3q22.3	27.7-27.9		2	Present in lung, gastrointestinal tract
CLD19	1p34.2	22.0-23.2	Hypomagnese mia with ocular involvement	2	Knockout affects nerve conduction
CLD20	6q25	23.5			
CLD21	4q35.1	25.4			
CLD22	4q35.1	25.5			Intronless gene
CLD23	8p23.1	31.9			Expressed in germinal center B cells, stomach, placenta
CLD24	4q35.1	22.8			
CLD25	11q23.2				

Claudins 13, 26 and 27 are not found in humans

Table 1. Some characteristics of different claudins present in humans

end contains the PDZ domains by which scaffolding proteins like ZO1 and ZO2 attach to claudins (1, 12). The larger of the extracellular loops (EL1) influences paracellular charge selectivity and contains the co-receptor site for Hepatitis C virus (HCV) (1,12). The smaller loop (EL2) mediates attachment of the claudin molecule to the corresponding one of the neighbouring cell and also contains the oligomerisation site and receptor site for clostridium perfringens enterotoxin (CPE) (1,12) (Figure 1).

The larger loop (EL-1) regulates paracellular electrical and solute permeability. The smaller loop (EL-2) mediates attachment between claudins of different cells. Four transmembrane domains separate the ends of the loops from the intracellular sequences of the molecules. The intracellular carboxyterminal end contains attachment sites for the PDZ domains of ZO-1, ZO-2 and ZO-3 molecules. It also contains phosphorylation sites which influence the function of claudins.

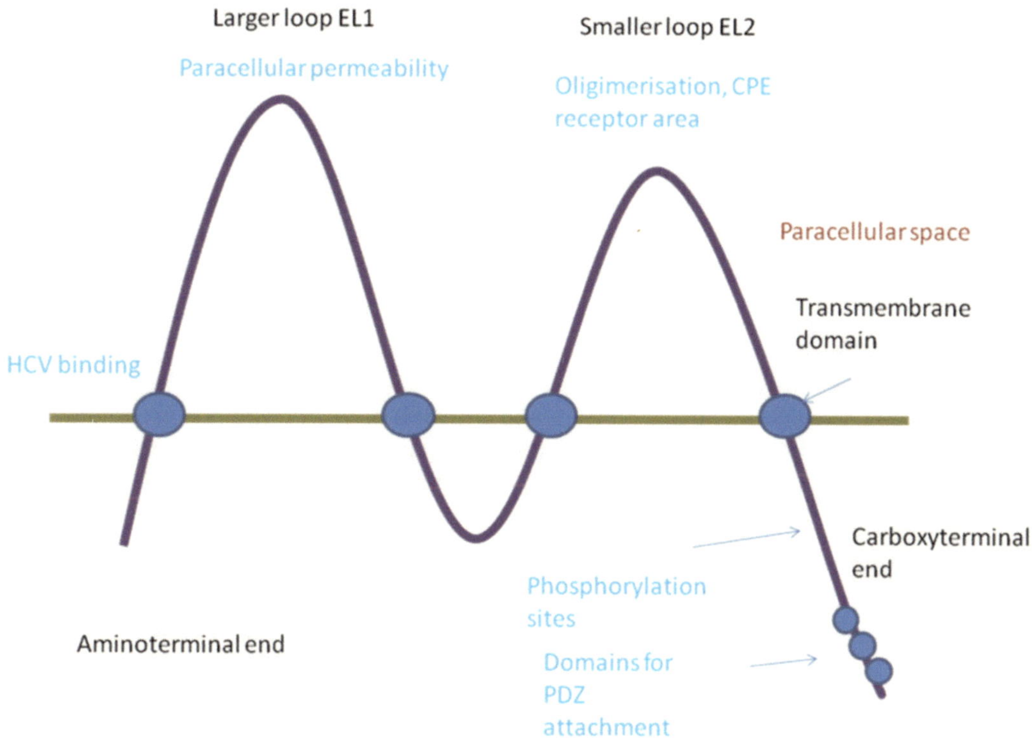

Fig. 1. A schematic presentation of the general molecular structure of claudins. Claudins form a structure formed by two extracellular loops (EL-1 and EL-2) in the cell membrane.

Claudins may associate with each other as homodimers or heterodimers (1). Heterodimerisation occurs selectively between specific claudins, for example, Claudins 1 can heterodimerise with 4 but not with 2 (1). In addition to such vertical association between neigbouring cells, claudins also bind to one another laterally on cell membranes to form the tight junctional strand (1). Claudin 2 expression in tight junctions generally leads to a leakier barrier function (1).Generally, claudins 2, 7, 10, 15 and 16 increase paracellular cation permeability by forming pores in the tight junctions whereas claudins 4, 5, 8, 11, 14 and 18 have an opposite function (1).

Claudins are widely expressed in epithelial cells but they are also found in endothelial and mesothelial cells, and in glial cells (2, 3, 13, 14). Several types of claudins are expressed in epithelial cells, but their distribution may vary according to the cell type and tissue site in question (2). Some claudins have a characteristic distribution. Claudin 5 is found in endothelial cells but it is also found in epithelium especially in neoplasia (1, 2). Claudin 11 is found in oligodendrocytes and in Sertoli cells but its expression has also been shown in endothelial cells of the corpus cavernosus (15, 16).

2.1 Claudins in disease

Claudin expression is modified in many diseases including both neoplastic and non-neoplastic conditions (5, 17). In cancers derived from epithelial cells claudin expression may be increased or decreased (17).The expression of claudins varies in tumors at different sites (7) and is different in head and neck (18), pancreatic (19), colonic (20,21), ovarian (22), and breast cancers (23) as well as within the same site like in gastric cancer, where there is lower expression of claudins in diffuse carcinoma compared to the intestinal type (24). In breast cancer claudin 4 expression is increased and its expression is found in more aggressive types of tumors (25). Claudin 16 expression, on the other hand, is associated with a better prognosis (26). Moreover, claudin 7 is downregulated in many cancers, such as breast and colon carcinoma, where its diminished expression is also associated with a poor prognosis (21, 27).

In non-epithelial cancers, claudin expression has been found in malignant mesotheliomas, tumors derived from cells lining serosal cavities (3). The expression of claudins is, however, lower than that found in epithelial tumors and the difference in claudin expression can be used in the differential diagnosis between mesotheliomas and adenocarcinomas metastatic to the lung (3). Such findings have been substantiated in many reports indicating that claudin 3 and 4 might be especially useful in this respect (3, 28).

Claudins may also be useful in the differential diagnosis between soft tissue tumors and carcinomas, especially when such tumors are poorly differentiated and their origin is hard to substantiate based on morphology alone. Soft tissue tumors generally do not express claudins, exceptions are synovial sarcomas which also morphologically contain epithelial elements, and perineurinomas (29, 30). Furthermore, hemangiomas and angiosarcomas express claudin 5, by which expression they can be distinguished from other soft tissue tumors (2).

In non-neoplastic diseases claudin expression may be deranged in diseases where the permeability of cell layers is disturbed. Such conditions include intestinal and kidney diseases, vascular diseases and lung diseases with a diminished or lost cellular permeability leading to tissue edema. In various inflammations, claudin expression may be deranged. Examples of such are chronic colitis, like Crohn's disease or colitis ulcerosa where expression of claudins have been changed (31,32). Many intestinal pathogens, such as aggressive strains of E coli, may lower the electrical and solute permeability of intestinal epithelia through displacement or downregulation of claudins and tight junctional scaffolding proteins leading to loss of fluid to the intestinal lumen (33,34). Claudins may also serve as receptors for bacterial toxins and viruses. Claudin 1 serves as a coreceptor for hepatitis virus 1, and several viruses may modify tight junctional permeability by downregulation or displacement of claudins from the tight junction (35, 36, 37, 38). Also bacterial toxins may use claudins as receptors. The toxin secreted by clostridium perfringens uses claudin 3 and 4 as receptors to open up paracellular spaces between cells (39). This also leads to cellular destruction and clostridium perfringens enterotoxins has been used in experimental models as a chemical to destroy ovarian and prostate cancer cells which have a high expression of claudins 3 and 4 (39). Additionally, modified clostridium perfringens enterotoxin (CPE) can be used in treatment of cancer to enable penetration of cytostatic drugs to cancer tissues (5, 39).

In the kidney, claudins are differentially expressed along the tubular segments leading to a modulated anionic and solute permeability in different regions of the segments which is detrimental for the absorption functions of the kidney (9). Claudins 16 and 19, for instance, regulate Mg and Cl permeability of the kidney tubular cells and mutations in these claudins lead to disturbances of the permeability of these electrolytes (40). In lung diseases like ARDS, expression of claudin 4 is downregulated leading to increased permeability of the alveolar wall (41, 42). Counteracting claudin 4 downregulation could thus be one putative treatment for this often fatal lung disease.

2.2 Claudins in gonadal structures

In mRNA and array analysis indicate that claudins 1, 2, 3, 5, 7, 8, 10, 11, 12, and 23 are present in testicular tissue of rodents. Claudin 11 is found to be the highest (15). Such studies do not, however, indicate the location of claudin mRNA, and claudin 5 mRNA, for instance, may also partly be derived from endothelial cells.

In human testicular tissues claudin 1, 6 and 7 protein expression has been found in seminiferous tubules (43). In rete testis epithelium, claudins 1 and 7 are strongly expressed while claudin 4 is weak and claudins 3, 5 and 6 are negative (43). Claudin 11 is present in Sertoli cells and takes part in formation of the blood testis barrier (44). In normal seminiferous epithelium claudin 11 is located at the basal compartment and the distribution is similar to ZO1 and ZO2 in this location (45). Claudin 1, 3 and 11 expression in Sertoli cells of mouse and rat testis appears to be regulated by androgens (46, 47, 48). Also gonadotropins regulate the expression of tight junctional proteins such as claudin 11 and occludin (49).

Expression of claudins and other tight junction proteins have not been studied in ovaries to such an extent as in the testis. Trace amounts of claudin 1, 2 , 4, 5, 7, 10, 11, 12 have been detected in normal ovarian tissues (17). Ovarian surface epithelial cells express claudin 1, ZO1 and occludin (50). Ovarian HOSE (human ovarian surface epithelial) cells do not express claudins 3 or 4 (51). On the other hand, in array based analysis, ovarian serous cancer cells displayed a strong mRNA expression of claudins 3, 4 and 7 compared to non-neoplastic cells (52).Claudin 3 and 4 expression appears to be nonexistent in surface ovarian cells but is increased in ovarian cysts (53).

3. Germ cell tumors

Germ cell tumors represent a tumor group derived from primordial germ cells of the body (54). They develop in testicular and ovarial tissues but are also found at extragonadal sites such as the mediastinum, and hypothalamic or suprasellar regions. Up to 95 % of testicular tumors are of germ cell derivation while in ovaries they make up only of 3-5 % of the tumor cases (55). Germ cell tumors of the testis develop from intratubular germ cell neoplasia (ITGCN) (except for spermatocytic seminoma and infantile germ cell tumors) and their development is linked to maturation arrest.The corresponding ovarian counterpart for ITGCN is gonadoblastoma (56).

Germ cell tumors can be divided in pure and mixed form (54). Pure germ cell tumors are composed of only one tumor component while mixed tumors consist of two or more (54). Testicular mixed germ cell tumors represent 30 to 50 % of the tumors while in the ovaries they represent about 20 %. The commonest pure germ cell tumor is seminoma/dysgerminoma representing 50 % and 40 % of testicular and ovarian germ cell tumors, respectively. Embryonal carcinoma is composed of undifferentiated cells with an epithelial appearance and it is more common in testis than in ovaries (54,57). Yolk sac tumor, on the other hand, is relatively more common in the ovaries (57). There are many histologic patterns, such as microcystic, papillary, macrocystic, hepatoid, solid and glandular-alveolar patterns, often mixed with each other (54). The tumor recapitulates the structures of yolk sac, the allantoin membrane and extraembryonic mesenchyme (54). It contains hyaline globules and Schiller-Duval bodies (57). Choriocarcinoma is rare both in ovaries and testis (54). It is composed of neoplastic cytotrophoblastic and syncytiotrophoblastic cells intermixed with hemorrhagic and necrotic background (54). Examples of benign germ cell tumors are teratomas which display a mixture of mature endodermal, mesodermal or ectodermal components (54). In some teratomas one component may predominate. Such is the case in dermoid cysts which contain a predominant component of cutaneous tissue leading to a cystic tumor containing keratin and hair structures (58). In immature teratomas or teratomas with somite type malignancies one or more components of the cell layers is malignant (54).

Immunohistochemical markers useful in the diagnosis of germ cell tumors include AFP and HCG which are positive in yolk sac tumor and choriocarcinoma, respectively (54,59). PLAP is invariably present in both but also in seminoma and embryonal carcinoma (54,59). They both express OCT3/4 which is not present in yolk sac tumor or choriocarcinoma (54,59). Embryonal carcinoma expresses SOX2 and CD30 which are not present in seminoma which, on the other hand, expresses SOX 17 (54,59).

4. Claudins in germ cell tumors

Germ cell tumors are neoplasms which are derived and may express several cell types of the ectoderm, endoderm or mesoderm. There are also many times a mixture of different cell components in these tumors (54). Of benign germ cell tumors a good example is teratoma which contains full developed components of epithelial, mesodermal and/or neural elements (54,58). Claudin expression in these tumors is analogous to the expression found in tissues of the comparable non-neoplastic tissues in human body (43). Thus expression of claudins 1, 2, 3, 4, 5 and 7 is usually amply found but expression is different in squamous or glandular epithelia (43). Squamous epithelium expresses strongly claudin 1 and 4 but claudin 3 is weakly or negatively expressed (43). On the other hand, glandular epithelia express claudin 3 strongly in teratomas (43). Claudin 7 is strongly expressed in both of these epithelia, but claudin 5 and 6 are negative (43). The different expression of claudins 3 and 4 is also reflected in malignant tumors derived from squamous or glandular epithelia. Adenocarcinomas of the oesophagus show a significantly higher expression of claudin 3 than squamous cell carcinomas (60). A similar situation is found for between lung squamous cell and adenocarcinomas (61). Mesenchymal tissues are generally negative for claudins with the exception of claudin 5 which is expressed in endothelial cells (2). Blood vessels may also show expression of some other claudins, like claudins 2 and 3 (2). Tissues found in teratomas are, however, many and strong conclusions cannot be drawn based on materials consisting only of some cases.

Teratocarcinomas express variable levels of claudins 1, 2, 3, 4 and 7 in carcinomatous elements but some cases display also positivity for claudins 5 and 6 (43). Claudin 5 which is mainly an endothelial marker and partly responsible for the function of blood brain or blood testis barrier (15, 62) is overexpressed in several carcinomas, like ovarian or lung carcinomas (61, 63, 64). The expression appears to be present in poorly differentiated tumors in serous ovarian carcinomas and is associated with a worse survival (64). Such expression may reflect a more primitive nature of the epithelial tumor cells but may also be an expression of vascular mimicry in tumors reflecting the capacity of neoplastic epithelial cells to attain endothelial features, a phenomenon described in melanomas, sarcomas and carcinomas (65,66). Whether expression of claudin 5 in teratocarcinomas influences behavior of these tumors is, however, unknown.

In tumor biology, derivation of malignant tumors has been suggested, on one hand, to clonal evolution of malignant cells, on the other hand, tumors have been suggested to develop through stem cells (67, 68). In clonal evolution there is a constant development of varied population of malignant cells and the most apt ones having the best survival capabilities to survive and make up the bulk of the tumors and develop metastases (67,68). According to the stem cell theory, tumors contain a population of stem cells which are present in specific locations (niche) in tumors (68). These cells which produce cancer tissue through dysregulation of asymmetric division are the basic invasive and metastasizing elements of the tumor and the rest are a more differentiated bulk which have not a significant impact on the spread and survival of the cells (68). Primitive pluripotent stem cells do not usually express antigens. Organ specific stem cells already committed to a specific differentiation can, however, be characterized by specific antigens (69). Such antigens present in breast carcinomas are CD44 and CD25, for instance (69). Of claudins, claudin 6 has been suggested to be an early epithelial stem cell marker (70). In line with this claudin 6 was present in a proportion of epithelial elements of teratocarcinomas, and in embryonal carcinomas but also in yolk sac or choriocarcinomatous elements suggesting that such claudin 6 positive stem cell may also differentiate towards extraembryonic cells (43).

Generally, however, claudins are parts of an element which is a sign of differentiation in epithelia, and their presence on the cell membrane of epithelia speaks for the presence of functioning tight junctions (1,2). Thus, a feature expected for a stem cells could be a lack of claudin expression. Indeed, in breast carcinoma, a claudin low population of breast carcinomas, having a low expression of claudins 3, 4 and 7 has been characterized to represent a tumor with similar features to the triple negative breast tumors and having a significant overlap with them (71). Even though there is a diminished expression of claudin 3 and 4 in embryonal carcinoma and claudin 3 in teratocarcinoma, both tumors express strongly claudin 7 and generally express claudins 1-7. The concept of stem cells cannot thus be addressed through diminished or absent claudin expression in germ cell tumors.

Embryonal carcinomas are primitive tumors committed to the epithelial lineage. In line with this they express claudins 1-7 (43). There is only one study which has investigated claudin expression in these tumors, but work has also been carried out in embryonal carcinoma cell lines. In the studies of Sawada et al, the F9 embryonal carcinoma cell line expressed the studied claudins 6 and 7 and this expression was induced by hepatocyte nuclear factor alpha (72). It also induced the formation of tight junctions and a polarised morphology of these cells and retarded cellular proliferation by upregulation p21 (72). Differentiation of embryonal cells to embryoid bodies increase the mRNA of several claudins, such as claudins 2, 6 and 7 and also occludin (73).

Seminomas are primitive germ cell tumors which have a specific morphology consisting of nests of large round cells which are usually surrounded by an inflammatory infiltrate consisting of small lymphocytes (54). Seminomas express strongly claudin 7 but some cases express also claudin 5 (43). The specific expression of these claudins in seminomas with lack of claudins 3, 4 and 1 clearly distinguishes these tumors from other germ cell tumors (43). Seminomas also display a strong expression of twist suggesting that it might be one factor contributing to the lack of expression of these claudins (43). Twist expression is associated with a poor prognosis in some tumors, such as breast carcinoma, but generally the expression of twist is low in carcinomas (74). It, however, is supposed to contribute to epitheliomesenchymal transition (EMT) in organ specific tumors which is also in line with the association with this function (74). A high expression of twist in seminomas probably signifies an inherent character of these tumor cells to express this transcription factor and it probably has another function in such a non-epithelial neoplasm. There are, however, no clinical studies assessing the prognostic value of twist or claudins in seminoma or other germ cell tumors.

Choriocarcinomas are aggressive tumors differentiating towards trophoblastic cells (54). Areas of choriocarcinoma are many times present in mixed germ cell tumors and pure choriocarcinomas are rare (54). They consist of large, neoplastic trophoblastic cells with areas of strong hemorrhage (54). Choriocarcinoma cells have an especially strong expression of claudin 4 (43). Claudin 4 is commonly present in epithelial neoplasms and in several tissues and it is considered to have a sealing function on paracellular membranes (1). In lung diseases, for instance, claudin 4 is downregulated in acute respiratory distress syndrome and lung inflammations contributing to the development of lung edema (41,42). Claudin 4 also serves as a receptor for clostridium perfringens enterotoxin, and chemically modified enterotoxins have been used in cancer treatment to facilitate penetration of chemotherapeutics to claudin 4 positive tumors (39). The significance of the strong expression of claudin 4 in choriocarcinoma cells is obscure but suggests that its expression may be important for the function of trophoblastic cells.

Intratubular germ cell neoplasia is the precursor lesion of germ cell neoplasms of the testis (54). In studies on claudin 11 expression in these lesions, claudin 11 expression was increased but the increased did not take place in the neoplastic germ cells but in Sertoli cells where claudin 11 was displaced from the membrane (45). The relative protein expression of claudins 1-7 in testicular germ cell neoplasia and testicular tissue is presented in Table 2 (43).

Germ cell tumor component	claudin 1	claudin 3	claudin 4	claudin 5	claudin 6	claudin 7	
seminoma	-	-	-	++	-	++	
embryonal carcinoma	++	+	+	++	++	+++	
teratocarcinoma	+++	+	+++	++	++	+++	
teratoma	+++	++	+++	++	++	+++	
chorioncarcinoma	-	-	++	+	+	+	
Testicular tissue							
seminiferous tubules	+	-	-	-	+	+	
Rete testis epithelium	+++	-	+	-	-	+++	

-=negative; += weak, ++= moderate, +++= strong expression

Table 2. Summary of the average protein expression of claudins 1, 3, 4, 5, 6 and 7 in germ cell tumors and testicular tissues

5. Claudins in diagnosis and treatment of germ cell tumors

Seminomas differ from other germ cell tumors by their expression of claudin 5 and 7 and lack of other claudins (43). Choriocarcinoma, on the other hand, expresses claudin 4 strongly (43). However, germ cell tumors have a specific histopathologic character and many times it is easy to distinguish seminoma or chorioncarcinoma from other germ cell tumors. In lymph node metastases, analysis of claudins might be of some help. Seminomas in lymphatic tissues in the mediastinum, for instance, may resemble the syncytial variant of nodular sclerosis Hodgkin's disease which do not express claudins at all (2). Germ cell tumors, however, have already established markers and claudins may hardly will be of any additional help in their diagnosis (54).

Claudins 3 and 4 have been found to function as receptors for clostridium perfringens enterotoxin (CPE) (39). In prostate and ovarian cancer cell lines expressing claudins 3 and 4 clostridium perfringens enterotoxin is able to destroy such cells (75,76). Claudins 3 and 4 are, however, expressed in many non-neoplastic cells so CPE cannot be used in treatment of cancer without side effects even though the cytotoxicity appears to be lower in non-neoplastic cells (76). Chemically modified CPE has, however, been used to open up tight junctions in cancer treatment experiments to allow a better penetrance of chemotherapeutic drugs to reach cancer cells (77). Such treatments strategy might also be possible in intratubular germ cell neoplasia when the tumor cells are still enveloped by the blood testis barrier. The main claudin responsible for the tight junctional permeability in the blood testis barrier is claudin 11, although claudins 3 and 5 also play some role (15). Additionally, CPE treatment based on cytotoxicity might be theoretically possible in those cases of germ cell neoplasia expressing claudins 3 and 4, like chorioncarcinoma or embryonal carcinoma (43).

5.1 Claudins in Sertoli cells

The blood testis barrier is formed by tight junctions between adjacent Sertoli cells (15). Claudin 11 is obligatory for the function and formation of tight junctional barrier in the testis (15). In claudin 11 knockout mice, Sertoli cells are detached from the seminiferous tubules and attain fibroblastoid features (78). In androgen receptor depleted mice the development of tight junctions of Sertoli cells is deranged with aberrations in the expression of several genes including occludin, claudin 11 and 3 (79, 80). Additionally, also claudin 5 mRNA has been detected in seminiferous epithelial cells and its expression is increased in mice at the time of blood testis barrier development (15). The expression of claudin 5 was dependent on ets variant gene 5 (ETV5) and germ cells (15). Interestingly, claudin 5 was not affected by ETV5 in vascular structures of the testis (15). The loss of claudin 5 expression in Sertoli cells resulted in an elevated solute permeability as detected by biotin tracer leakage (15).

TGFbeta3 inhibits the expression of claudin 11, occludin and ZO1 by a MAP 38 kinase dependent mechanism in Sertoli cells (81). FSH and TNF alpha inhibits claudin 11 expression in Sertoli cell culture (82). Testosterone increases claudin 11 mRNA expression in a dose dependent manner (47). The influence of antiandrogenic flutamide is complex (47). Fetally administered flutamide in mice resulted in prepubertal decrease of claudin 11 in Sertoli cells but the inhibition in adult testes was dose dependent, lower doses resulting in decreased expression (47). When given orally to 13 weeks' old rats, flutamide induced a decrease in the mRNA expression of occludin but did not affect claudin 1 or 11 mRNA (83). Thus androgens and gonadotropins may theoretically influence the penetrance of the blood testis barrier by modifying claudin 11 expression but such treatment strategy may lead to intolerable side effects perhaps through breakage of self tolerance and development of autoimmune diseases or reactions induced by exposure of self antigens normally hidden by the blood testis barrier.

6. References

[1] Krause G, Winkler L, Mueller SL, Haseloff RF, Piontek J, Blasig IE: Structure and function of claudins. Biochim Biophys Acta. 2008, 1778: 631-45

[2] Soini Y. Expression of claudins 1, 2, 3, 4, 5 and 7 in various types of tumours. Histopathology 2005;46:551-60.

[3] Soini Y, Kinnula V, Kahlos K, Pääkkö P: Claudins in differential diagnosis between mesothelioma and metastatic adenocarcinoma of the pleura. J Clin Pathol. 2006, 59: 250-4.

[4] Sawada N, Murata M, Kikuchi K, Osanai M, Tobioka H, Kojima T, Chiba H: Tightjunctions and human diseases. Med Electron Microsc. 2003, 36: 147-56.

[5] Soini Y. Claudins in lung diseases. Respir Res. 2011 May 27;12:70.

[6] Godfrey RW: Human airway epithelial tight junctions. Microsc Res Tech. 1997, 38: 488-99.

[7] Matter K, Balda MS. Epithelial tight junctions, gene expression and nucleo-junctional interplay. J Cell Sci. 2007, 120: 1505-11.

[8] Mineta K, Yamamoto Y, Yamazaki Y, Tanaka H, Tada Y, Saito K, Tamura A, Igarashi M, Endo T, Takeuchi K, Tsukita S. Predicted expansion of the claudin multigene family. FEBS Lett. 2011, 585:606-12.

[9] Kirk A, Campbell S, Bass P, Mason J, Collins J. Differential expression of claudin tight junction proteins in the human cortical nephron. Nephrol Dial Transplant. 2010;25:2107-19.

[10] Holmes JL, Van Itallie CM, Rasmussen JE, Anderson JM. Claudin profiling in the mouse during postnatal intestinal development and along the gastrointestinal tract reveals complex expression patterns. Gene Expr Patterns. 2006;6:581-8.

[11] Hartsock A, Nelson WJ. Adherens and tight junctions: structure, function and connections to the actin cytoskeleton. Biochim Biophys Acta. 2008;1778:660-9.

[12] Lal-Nag M, Morin PJ: The claudins. Genome Biol. 2009, 10: 235.

[13] Mack AF, Wolburg H. Growing axons in fish optic nerve are accompanied by astrocytes interconnected by tight junctions. Brain Res. 2006;1103:25-31.

[14] Tiwari-Woodruff SK, Buznikov AG, Vu TQ, Micevych PE, Chen K, Kornblum HI, Bronstein JM. OSP/claudin-11 forms a complex with a novel member of the tetraspanin super family and beta1 integrin and regulates proliferation and migration of oligodendrocytes. J Cell Biol. 2001;153:295-305.

[15] Morrow CM, Mruk D, Cheng CY, Hess RA. Claudin and occludin expression and function in the seminiferous epithelium. Philos Trans R Soc Lond B Biol Sci. 2010;365:1679-96.

[16] Wessells H, Sullivan CJ, Tsubota Y, Engel KL, Kim B, Olson NE, Thorner D, Chitaley K. Transcriptional profiling of human cavernosal endothelial cells reveals distinctive cell adhesion phenotype and role for claudin 11 in vascular barrier function. Physiol Genomics. 2009;39:100-8.

[17] Hewitt KJ, Agarwal R, Morin PJ. The claudin gene family: expression in normal and neoplastic tissues. BMC Cancer. 2006;6:186.

[18] Al Moustafa AE, aoui-Jamali MA, Batist G, Hernandez-Perez M, Serruya C, Alpert L, Black MJ, Sladek R, Foulkes WD. Identification of genes associated with head and neck carcinogenesis by cDNA microarray comparison between matched primary normal epithelial and squamous carcinoma cells. Oncogene 2002;21:2634-2640.

[19] Tsukahara M, Nagai H, Kamiakito T, Kawata H, Takayashiki N, Saito K, Tanaka A. Distinct expression patterns of claudin-1 and claudin-4 in intraductal papillary-mucinous tumors of the pancreas. Pathol Int 2005;55:63-69.

[20] Kinugasa T, Huo Q, Higashi D, Shibaguchi H, Kuroki M, Tanaka T, Futami K, Yamashita Y, Hachimine K, Maekawa S, Nabeshima K, Iwasaki H, Kuroki M. Selective up-regulation of claudin-1 and claudin-2 in colorectal cancer. Anticancer Res 2007;27:3729-3734.

[21] Oshima T, Kunisaki C, Yoshihara K, Yamada R, Yamamoto N, Sato T, Makino H, Yamagishi S, Nagano Y, Fujii S, Shiozawa M, Akaike M, Wada N, Rino Y, Masuda M, Tanaka K, Imada T. Reduced expression of the claudin-7 gene correlates with venous invasion and liver metastasis in colorectal cancer. Oncol Rep 2008;19:953-959.

[22] Agarwal R, D'Souza T, Morin PJ. Claudin-3 and claudin-4 expression in ovarian epithelial cells enhances invasion and is associated with increased matrix metalloproteinase-2 activity. Cancer Res 2005;65:7378-7385.

[23] Sauer T, Pedersen MK, Ebeltoft K, Naess O. Reduced expression of Claudin-7 in fine needle aspirates from breast carcinomas correlate with grading and metastatic disease. Cytopathology 2005;16:193-198.

[24] Soini Y, Tommola S, Helin H, Martikainen P. Claudins 1, 3, 4 and 5 in gastric carcinoma, loss of claudin expression associates with the diffuse subtype. Virchows Arch 2006;448:52-58.

[25] Lanigan F, McKiernan E, Brennan DJ, Hegarty S, Millikan RC, McBryan J, Jirstrom K, Landberg G, Martin F, Duffy MJ, Gallagher WM. Increased claudin-4 expression is associated with poor prognosis and high tumour grade in breast cancer. Int J Cancer. 2009;124:2088-97.

[26] Martin TA, Harrison GM, Watkins G, Jiang WG. Claudin-16 reduces the aggressive behavior of human breast cancer cells. J Cell Biochem. 2008;105:41-52.

[27] Sauer T, Pedersen MK, Ebeltoft K, Naess O. Reduced expression of Claudin-7 in fine needle aspirates from breast carcinomas correlate with grading and metastatic disease. Cytopathology. 2005;16:193-8.

[28] Facchetti F, Gentili F, Lonardi S, Bercich L, Santin A. Claudin-4 in mesothelioma diagnosis. Histopathology. 2007, 51: 261-3.

[29] Billings SD, Walsh SV, Fisher C, Nusrat A, Weiss SW, Folpe AL. Aberrant expression of tight junction-related proteins ZO-1, claudin-1 and occludin in synovial sarcoma: an immunohistochemical study with ultrastructural correlation. Mod Pathol. 2004;17:141-9.

[30] Folpe AL, Billings SD, McKenney JK, Walsh SV, Nusrat A, Weiss SW. Expression of claudin-1, a recently described tight junction-associated protein, distinguishes soft tissue perineurioma from potential mimics. Am J Surg Pathol. 2002;26:1620-6.

[31] Zeissig S, Bürgel N, Günzel D, Richter J, Mankertz J, Wahnschaffe U, Kroesen AJ, Zeitz M, Fromm M, Schulzke JD. Changes in expression and distribution of claudin 2, 5 and 8 lead to discontinuous tight junctions and barrier dysfunction in active Crohn's disease. Gut. 2007;56:61-72.

[32] Oshima T, Miwa H, Joh T. Changes in the expression of claudins in active ulcerative colitis. J Gastroenterol Hepatol. 2008;23:S146-50.

[33] Hering NA, Richter JF, Krug SM, Günzel D, Fromm A, Bohn E, Rosenthal R, Bücker R, Fromm M, Troeger H, Schulzke JD: Yersinia enterocolitica induces epithelial barrier dysfunction through regional tight junction changes in colonic HT-29/B6 cell monolayers. Lab Invest. 2011, 91: 310-324

[34] Strauman MC, Harper JM, Harrington SM, Boll EJ, Nataro JP: Enteroaggregative Escherichia coli disrupts epithelial cell tight junctions. Infect Immun. 2010, 78: 4958-64.

[35] Evans MJ, von Hahn T, Tscherne DM, Syder AJ, Panis M, Wölk B, Hatziioannou T, McKeating JA, Bieniasz PD, Rice CM: Claudin-1 is a hepatitis C virus co-receptor required for a late step in entry. Nature. 2007, 446: 801-5.

[36] Yeo NK, Jang YJ: Rhinovirus infection-induced alteration of tight junction and adherens junction components in human nasal epithelial cells. Laryngoscope. 2010, 120: 346-52.

[37] Nazli A, Chan O, Dobson-Belaire WN, Ouellet M, Tremblay MJ, Gray-Owen SD, Arsenault AL, Kaushic C: Exposure to HIV-1 directly impairs mucosal epithelial barrier integrity allowing microbial translocation. PLoS Pathog. 2010, 6: e1000852

[38] Nava P, López S, Arias CF, Islas S, González-Mariscal L: The rotavirus surface protein VP8 modulates the gate and fence function of tight junctions in epithelial cells. J Cell Sci. 2004, 117: 5509-19.

[39] Van Itallie CM, Betts L, Smedley JG 3rd, McClane BA, Anderson JM: Structure of the claudin-binding domain of Clostridium perfringens enterotoxin. J Biol Chem. 2008, 283: 268-74.

[40] Hou J, Renigunta A, Gomes AS, Hou M, Paul DL, Waldegger S, Goodenough DA. Claudin-16 and claudin-19 interaction is required for their assembly into tight junctions and for renal reabsorption of magnesium. Proc Natl Acad Sci U S A. 2009;106:15350-5.

[41] Wray C, Mao Y, Pan J, Chandrasena A, Piasta F, Frank JA: Claudin-4 augments alveolar epithelial barrier function and is induced in acute lung injury. Am J Physiol Lung Cell Mol Physiol. 2009, 297: L219-27.

[42] Xia XM, Wang FY, Wang ZK, Wan HJ, Xu WA, Lu H: Emodin enhances alveolar epithelial barrier function in rats with experimental acute pancreatitis. World J Gastroenterol. 2010, 16: 2994-3001.

[43] Väre P, Soini Y. Twist is inversely associated with claudins in germ cell tumors of the testis. APMIS. 2010;118(9):640-7

[44] Bronstein JM, Chen K, Tiwari-Woodruff S, Kornblum HI. Developmental expression of OSP/claudin-11. J Neurosci Res. 2000;60:284-90.

[45] Fink C, Weigel R, Fink L, Wilhelm J, Kliesch S, Zeiler M, Bergmann M, Brehm R. Claudin-11 is over-expressed and dislocated from the blood-testis barrier in Sertoli cells associated with testicular intraepithelial neoplasia in men. Histochem Cell Biol. 2009;131:755-64.

[46] Gye MC. Expression of claudin-1 in mouse testis. Arch Androl. 2003;49:271-9..

[47] Florin A, Maire M, Bozec A, Hellani A, Chater S, Bars R, Chuzel F, Benahmed M. Androgens and postmeiotic germ cells regulate claudin-11 expression in rat Sertoli cells. Endocrinology. 2005;146:1532-40.

[48] Meng J, Holdcraft RW, Shima JE, Griswold MD, Braun RE. Androgens regulate the permeability of the blood-testis barrier. Proc Natl Acad Sci U S A. 2005;102:16696-700.

[49] McCabe MJ, Tarulli GA, Meachem SJ, Robertson DM, Smooker PM, Stanton PG. Gonadotropins regulate rat testicular tight junctions in vivo. Endocrinology. 2010;151:2911-22.

[50] Zhu Y, Maric J, Nilsson M, Brännström M, Janson PO, Sundfeldt K. Formation and barrier function of tight junctions in human ovarian surface epithelium. Biol Reprod. 2004;71:53-9.

[51] Agarwal R, D'Souza T, Morin PJ. Claudin-3 and claudin-4 expression in ovarian epithelial cells enhances invasion and is associated with increased matrix metalloproteinase-2 activity. Cancer Res. 2005;65:7378-85.

[52] Santin AD, Zhan F, Bellone S, Palmieri M, Cane S, Bignotti E, Anfossi S, Gokden M, Dunn D, Roman JJ, O'Brien TJ, Tian E, Cannon MJ, Shaughnessy J Jr, Pecorelli S. Gene expression profiles in primary ovarian serous papillary tumors and normal ovarian epithelium: identification of candidate molecular markers for ovarian cancer diagnosis and therapy. Int J Cancer. 2004;112:14-25.

[53] Zhu Y, Brännström M, Janson PO, Sundfeldt K. Differences in expression patterns of the tight junction proteins,claudin 1, 3, 4 and 5, in human ovarian surface epithelium as compared to epithelia in inclusion cysts and epithelial ovarian tumours. Int J Cancer. 2006;118:1884-91.

[54] Eble J, Sauter G, Epstein JI, Sesterhenn IA. Tumours of the Urinary system and Male Genital Organs, WHO Classification of Tumours. Lyon, France, 2004.

[55] Huyghe E, Matsuda T, Thonneau P. Increasing incidence of testicular cancer worldwide: a review. J Urol. 2003;170:5-11.

[56] Mancilla EE, Poggi H, Repetto G, Rumié H, García H, Ugarte F, Hidalgo S, Jara A, Muzzo S, Panteón E, Torrealba I, Foradori A, Cattani A. Y chromosome sequences in Turner's syndrome: association with virilization and gonadoblastoma. J Pediatr Endocrinol Metab. 2003;16:1157-63.

[57] Roth LM, Talerman A. Recent advances in the pathology and classification of ovarian germ cell tumors. Int J Gynecol Pathol. 2006;25:305-20.

[58] Tavassoli FA, Devilee P: Tumours of the breast and Female genital Organs. World Health Organization Classification of Tumours. IARC press, Lyon, France, 2003.

[59] Looijenga LH. Human testicular (non)seminomatous germ cell tumours: the clinical implications of recent pathobiological insights. J Pathol. 2009;218:146-62.

[60] Takala H, Saarnio J, Wiik H, Soini Y. Claudins 1, 3, 4, 5 and 7 in esophageal cancer: loss of claudin 3 and 4 expression is associated with metastatic behavior. APMIS. 2007;115:838-47.

[61] Merikallio H, Kaarteenaho R, Pääkkö P, Lehtonen S, Hirvikoski P, Mäkitaro R, Harju T, Soini Y. Impact of smoking on the expression of claudins in lung carcinoma. Eur J Cancer. 2011;47:620-30.

[62] Nitta T, Hata M, Gotoh S, Seo Y, Sasaki H, Hashimoto N, Furuse M, Tsukita S.Size-selective loosening of the blood-brain barrier in claudin-5-deficient mice. J Cell Biol. 2003;161:653-60.

[63] Soini Y, Talvensaari-Mattila A. Expression of claudins 1, 4, 5, and 7 in ovarian tumors of diverse types. Int J Gynecol Pathol. 2006;25:330-5.

[64] Turunen M, Talvensaari-Mattila A, Soini Y, Santala M. Claudin-5 overexpression correlates with aggressive behavior in serous ovarian adenocarcinoma. Anticancer Res. 2009;29:5185-9.
[65] Hendrix MJ, Seftor EA, Hess AR, Seftor RE. Vasculogenic mimicry and tumour-cell plasticity: lessons from melanoma. Nat Rev Cancer. 2003;3:411-21.
[66] Folberg R, Maniotis AJ. Vasculogenic mimicry. APMIS. 2004;112:508-25.
[67] Barrett JC. Mechanisms of multistep carcinogenesis and carcinogen risk assessment. Environ Health Perspect. 1993;100:9-20.
[68] Sell S. On the stem cell origin of cancer. Am J Pathol. 2010;176:2584-494.
[69] Fábián A, Barok M, Vereb G, Szöllosi J. Die hard: are cancer stem cells the Bruce Willises of tumor biology? Cytometry A. 2009;75(1):67-74.
[70] Turksen K, Troy TC. Claudin-6: a novel tight junction molecule is developmentally regulated in mouse embryonic epithelium. Dev Dyn. 2001;222:292-300.
[71] Prat A, Parker JS, Karginova O, Fan C, Livasy C, Herschkowitz JI, He X, Perou CM. Phenotypic and molecular characterization of the claudin-low intrinsic subtype of breast cancer. Breast Cancer Res. 2010;12:R68
[72] Chiba H, Gotoh T, Kojima T, Satohisa S, Kikuchi K, Osanai M, Sawada N. Hepatocyte nuclear factor (HNF)-4alpha triggers formation of functional tight junctions and establishment of polarized epithelial morphology in F9 embryonal carcinoma cells. Exp Cell Res. 2003;286:288-97.
[73] Guillemot L, Hammar E, Kaister C, Ritz J, Caille D, Jond L, Bauer C, Meda P, Citi S. Disruption of the cingulin gene does not prevent tight junction formation but alters gene expression. J Cell Sci. 2004;117:5245-56.
[74] Soini Y, Tuhkanen H, Sironen R, Virtanen I, Kataja V, Auvinen P, Mannermaa A, Kosma VM. Transcription factors zeb1, twist and snai1 in breast carcinoma. BMC Cancer. 2011;11:73.
[75] Yuan X, Lin X, Manorek G, Kanatani I, Cheung LH, Rosenblum MG, Howell SB. Recombinant CPE fused to tumor necrosis factor targets human ovarian cancer cells expressing the claudin-3 and claudin-4 receptors. Mol Cancer Ther. 2009;8:1906-15.
[76] Maeda T, Murata M, Chiba H, Takasawa A, Tanaka S, Kojima T, Masumori N, Tsukamoto T, Sawada N. Claudin-4-targeted therapy using Clostridium perfringens enterotoxin for prostate cancer. Prostate. 2011[Epub ahead of print]
[77] Kondoh M, Takahashi A, Fujii M, Yagi K, Watanabe Y. A novel strategy for a drug delivery system using a claudin modulator. Biol Pharm Bull. 2006;29:1783-9.
[78] Mazaud-Guittot S, Meugnier E, Pesenti S, Wu X, Vidal H, Gow A, Le Magueresse-Battistoni B. Claudin 11 deficiency in mice results in loss of the Sertoli cell epithelial phenotype in the testis. Biol Reprod. 2010;82:202-13.
[79] Wang RS, Yeh S, Chen LM, Lin HY, Zhang C, Ni J, Wu CC, di Sant'Agnese PA, deMesy-Bentley KL, Tzeng CR, Chang C. Androgen receptor in sertoli cell is essential for germ cell nursery and junctional complex formation in mouse testes. Endocrinology. 2006;147:5624-33.

[80] Willems A, Batlouni SR, Esnal A, Swinnen JV, Saunders PT, Sharpe RM, França LR, De Gendt K, Verhoeven G. Selective ablation of the androgen receptor in mouse sertoli cells affects sertoli cell maturation, barrier formation and cytoskeletal development. PLoS One. 2010;5:e14168.

[81] Lui WY, Lee WM, Cheng CY. Transforming growth factor-beta3 perturbs the inter-Sertoli tight junction permeability barrier in vitro possibly mediated via its effects on occludin, zonula occludens-1, and claudin-11. Endocrinology. 200;142:1865-77.

[82] Hellani A, Ji J, Mauduit C, Deschildre C, Tabone E, Benahmed M. Developmental and hormonal regulation of the expression of oligodendrocyte-specific protein/claudin 11 in mouse testis. Endocrinology. 2000;141:3012-9.

[83] Gye MC, Ohsako S. Effects of flutamide in the rat testis on the expression of occludin, an integral member of the tight junctions. Toxicol Lett. 2003;143:217-22.